The Father Trimester:

The Pivotal Role of the Black Father in Breastfeeding

Bamidele Best
Introduction by Naila Best

Copyright © 2022 Xavier Best
All rights reserved.
ISBN- 9798439544899

Dedicated to my amazing wife Naila, my eldest son Mikey, and our beloved ancestor Dr. Llaila O. Afrika. Most importantly, this book was written in tribute to and as a gift to our newborn son Jahi. Your joyful presence is a daily reminder of the spiritual mission we are charged with accomplishing for the total liberation of all Afrikan people. May this book be a source of inspiration and wisdom for you in your older years. Ase!

"It takes a breast for a child to know its mother and it takes a mother for a child to know its father."
-Afrikan Proverb

TABLE OF CONTENTS

ACKNOWLEDGMENTS

I would like to offer a heartfelt Asante Sana to the Creator for allowing me the mental and psychological space to produce this vision for my family and my people, my beautifully divine wife for patiently working with me with constructive critiques and insight to help make this the best book possible, and my son Mikey for providing me with the inspiration to embrace fatherhood with all its joys and challenges. I also would like to thank the Republic of Tanzania for providing a real home for my family after so many years in captivity and Mama Rose (Shangazi) and Dada Mwajuma for your abundance of generosity in caring for our family and newborn son in his first month of life. We would like to thank Dada Aleshi and Family for being our home away from home in Tanzania and always having the time to share your thoughts and counsel for the betterment of my family. You are truly our Mwalimu. Asante sana to Dada Dawah, Kaka Innocent and family for entrusting us to be your neighbors and consistently opening your home to our family, surrounding us with the positivity that has fueled our growth. Asante sana to our doula Osun Wunmi who despite geographic distance was able to effectively coach us through the prenatal and labor process so that our son could arrive safely. You are a true spiritual asset to our people. Asante to Fungi Dube for sharing your artistic vision with us to bring the cover design for this book to life. We are so grateful. Asante for Natina and Diallo for being Jahi's godparents and doing so much to facilitate the completion of this book. Last but certainly not least I would like to thank our son Jahi. Your arrival into this world has revitalized our family and renewed our mission to promote the liberation of our people worldwide. We vow to continue to make sacrifices on your behalf and pour into your spiritual growth and development. We love you!

P.S. Also thank you Jahi for making sure Mama's milk never runs dry.

— Baba Jahi

INTRODUCTION

When I first met my husband, I knew he was born for fatherhood. As a single mother of a seven-year-old at the time, I was raising a young boy in america with very little guidance or reassurance if I was doing it right. I was severely unaware of how crucial my role was as a mother. More importantly, I was naïve to the natural healing power that the divine father brings to the mother. Once I learned of its significance, I knew if I was awarded the opportunity of wifehood and motherhood, I would cherish & embody the roles at all costs.

Having a knowledgeable & caring Black man in my life was a game changer for me. His strong-willed yet gentle presence evolved me as a woman, but more importantly as a mother. As we set on our journey to become healthier, more involved parents in a society that demonizes holistic family practices, we quickly realized how isolating the journey was becoming. We faced a large amount of opposition from family and friends, but we were determined to stay the course since we knew we weren't just doing this for the health of our family, but for the health and preservation of ALL Black families.

This book was birthed out of our desire to holistically dispel the lies and misconceptions of western parenting practices, encourage the black community in america to reclaim the destiny of our families, in addition to restoring the necessity of the presence of the Black fathers' role in rearing whole, bonded children.

Through this book, Baba Bamidele brings to light the degenerate and death-centered history of european culture in regards to pregnancy, birth, and child rearing. He analyzes western medicine practices through a psychosocial lens, while juxtaposing those practices with the life-centered ways and culture of our Afrikan ancestors. He discusses the Black fathers' responsibility in safeguarding the mental & emotional growth of his family, as well as practical bonding techniques they can utilize. Black fathers will learn how to successfully encourage their wives through the breastfeeding journey, their role in the spiritual protection of the mother, preventable measures to take to combat postpartum depression in their partners, and so much more.

As a Black couple going through the beautiful transition into parenthood, we both saw a lack of information when it came to the importance of the Black father in promoting the emotional and

9

psychological stability of the Black mother. The power of this book, is that it was strictly constructed with Black people in mind. Although he largely focuses on the father's role, this book is useful to mothers as well, as it brings added clarity with regard to the do's and don'ts of the prenatal and postpartum periods, and will instill in both the mother and father a newfound knowledge and confidence in the realms of pregnancy, birth and beyond. This book is NOT for those who are deeply wedded to western ideals of health, medicine or parenting. If you fall into any of those categories, please read no further.

Historically parenthood has always been more than just a title, but something we embody. This is even shown in the customary practice of addressing mothers and fathers as "Mama" and "Baba" respectively followed by the first name of their children. It is through these prestigious roles that we assert our sacred responsibility to create the type of nations and cultures conducive to our long-term survival as a people. The Father Trimester is our libation to that revolutionary vision for the born and unborn. ASÉ

— Mama Jahi

PREFACE

The genesis of *The Father Trimester* arose from two urgent concerns: one, the continued psychological deterioration of Black people under the social, economic, and political domination of the United States and two, the successful, unassisted delivery of our first child together. These two events sparked my desire to become an advocate for other Black fathers to experience this level of power of which we've been robbed. I intuitively knew that the battles that we faced as a global Afrikan population were spiritual in nature and therefore the counterattack had to be equally spiritual in character.

After much research and internal searching I arrived at the conclusion that we would never experience true liberation as a people until we seized control of the birthing process. Relinquishing the power of childbirth to white people, our natural enemies, struck me as absurd on its face. How could we reasonably argue the divinity of Black children while simultaneously forfeiting this most sacred of rituals to those intent on our genetic destruction? Answering these questions called for radical action.

In addition to birthing our child on the African continent, my wife and I were determined to give birth at home in the most holistic setting possible. It was through this decision that we aspired to honor both our people and our ancestors.

As a father, I think it is imperative that we reclaim our role as militant protectors of the lives of our wives and children. This will mean a fundamental reorganization of entrenched beliefs and prejudices that have blocked us from manifesting the revolutionary masculine power to balance the feminine power of our women. In this regard, *The Father Trimester* must be properly understood as a spiritual call to arms for Black fathers to reassert ownership over our children and (by connection) our families and collective destiny.

The first chapter will address, in short form, the ancient and modern history of breastfeeding, its social, spiritual, and economic meanings as well as why it is critical we know this history. Chapter two will review the father's role in breastfeeding, the remarkable health benefits of Black mother's milk, and its central role as a psychological base for the long term mental and physical development of our children. Chapter three will explore the significance of home birth as an alternative to conventional, westernized hospital births while chapter four will detail the beauty of lotus birth and its indispensable role in providing a nutritional foundation for our baby's health. Chapters five through nine will expand upon preventive measures against postpartum depression, dietary recommendations for lactation, how to take advantage of community resources, and the intricate bonding techniques that fathers can adopt to nurture a biochemical connection with their newborn. Finally, chapters ten through thirteen will explain the tangible benefits of natural birth over unnatural birth, the necessity for maternity leave for fathers, the duty all fathers have to cultivate safe, life-centered environments (protecting the perimeter), and a redefinition of childbirth from a mere biological event to a spiritual rite of passage. This holistic approach to fatherhood aims to reignite a passion for childbirth and childrearing so that we may become true assets to our families and communities. More than any monetary or material reward our children will thank us in the form of functional, balanced relationships and nations. May we continue to grow into the teachers and elders the Creator intended us to be. Abibifahodie!

A clarification on the use of terms: throughout this book the term "Black" and "Afrikan" will be used interchangeably but in my living and research on the African continent I have come to the conclusion that Africa is the cultural cradle of all notions of health and wellness whereas "Black" is a term of relatively recent use to describe Afrikans in conditions of captivity (African Americans). Therefore, where the term "Black" appears it is used for the sake of convenience and not to overshadow the true historical origins of the practices elaborated upon in this book.

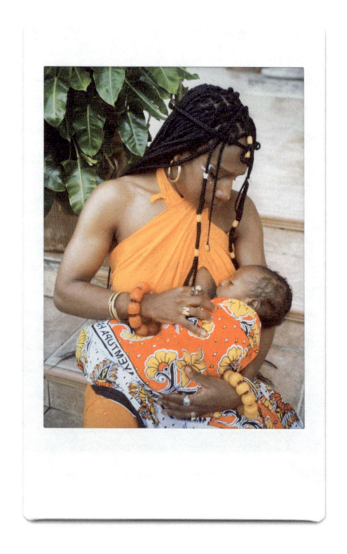

My wife breastfeeding Jahi

Chapter 1

A BRIEF HISTORY OF BREASTFEEDING

"Although God is often called Father in many regions, there is a significant tradition that presents God as Mother. In the Democratic Republic of Congo the Bakongo ethnic group, which still practices the matriarchal system, explicitly refers to God as 'Mother.' Elsewhere, God is referred to as 'Nursing Mother' (among the Maasai of Kenya and Tanzania), 'Great Mother' (Nuba of Sudan), 'Mother of People' (Ewe of Ghana, Benin, and Togo), and the 'Great Rainbow' (Chewa of Malawi and Zambia)."
—Mutumbo Nkulu-N'Sengha

The history of breastfeeding is as old as the history of humanity. It originated in the Great Lakes Region of inner Africa among the Twa people. Here family social dynamics relied upon the balanced application of male and female power or complementarity. The role and position of the woman was paramount in laying the foundation for not only family growth but societal evolution generally.

Further north, ancient artifacts reveal the significance of breastfeeding as a biological and spiritual reality in the Kingdom of Kush (Ethiopia). Metal and stone statues from 7th century (B.C.E.) Kemet exalted the divine mother Auset breastfeeding her son Heru in what art historians call the "lactan pose." It was the nourishing power of breastmilk that earned Auset the title of the Neter of Life-Giving Waters. Third Dynasty Kemetic multigenius and true father of medicine Imhotep published guidelines to facilitate breastfeeding in his Ebers Papyrus dated 1550 B.C.E., advising, "to get a supply of milk in a woman's breast for suckling a child," physicians must, "warm the bones of a sword fish in oil and rub her back with it. Or: Let the woman sit cross-legged and eat fragrant bread of soused durra, while rubbing her breasts with the poppy plant." It was only after the invasion of the Greeks in 332 B.C.E. that reliance on wet nurses and cow's milk came into wide use. Greeks such as Hippocrates even recommended giving infants honey and wine! Much of this history has been erased from living memory through a campaign cultural genocide led by Asian and European conquerors. Interestingly, a review of Greco-Roman myth reveals a culturally endemic practice of having animals breastfeed babies instead of humans. Numerous Greek and Roman "gods" are on record as having been nursed by animals in infancy[1]. The founders of Rome,

---

[1] An archeological excavation in Bavaria, Germany led by University of Bristol scientist J. Dunne uncovered spouted vessels dated from the Bronze Age with traces of animal milk inside. These vessels offer empirical evidence that Europeans were the first in the world to feed humans animal milk. *See* Dunne, J. et al. "Milk of Ruminants in Ceramic Baby Bottles from Prehistoric Child Graves." *Nature* 574, 246-248 (2019)

Romulus and Remus were suckled by a she-wolf; the Greek gods Zeus, Dionysus, and Asclepius were suckled by goats; Telephus by a deer, Hippothoon by a mare, and Hapis a pig. Justification for this bizarre practice was the belief that the characteristics of these wild animals was transmitted via the breastmilk to the baby (a lion transmitted courage and a wolf transmitted ravenousness). Incidentally, the frigid cold of northern, high-latitude climates—specifically those which characterized the Caucasus mountains during the Ice Age—likely complicated, if not eliminated, the possibility of breastfeeding for white women, making animal milk the only option. This deficiency of breast milk was due to the fact that, "a colder body temperature can slow down the body's milk ejection reflex."[2] Women with mastitis—an infection of the breast—also experience pain during breastfeeding which is aggravated under cold temperatures. Therefore, even a white mother with adequate milk supply who was able to avoid mastitis would experience pain during breastfeeding as an effect of cold temperatures on their nipples, problems Afrikan women never experienced thanks to the warm, equatorial environments in which they lived.

This reliance on animal wet nurses extended well beyond the realm of myth. In early industrial europe animals were routinely used as wet nurses for mothers who has been infected with syphilis. As University of Bologna scholar Giulia Perducci notes in his paper *Breastfeeding Animals and Other Wild 'Nurses' in Greek and Roman*

[2] Mack, Lindsay E. "BRRR: This Is How Cold Weather Affects Your Milk Supply and Ability to Breastfeed." *Romper*, Romper, 23 Nov. 2017, https://www.romper.com/p/how-cold-weather-affects-your-milk-supply-ability-to-breastfeed-2990585.

Mythology[3], "goats and donkeys were widely used to feed abandoned babies in hospitals in 18th and 19th century europe," and "suckling directly was preferable to milking an animal and drinking the milk, as contamination by microbes during the milking process could lead to the infant contracting deadly diarrheal diseases." Meanwhile, infant neglect was extremely common in Renaissance europe. Women in france were legally forced to breastfeed their babies for at least nine months in order to prevent them from abandoning their babies, which was a common practice for lactating women seeking employment in the growing wet nurse industry[4].

Wet nurses also figured prominently as a tactic to promote the genetic survival of whites during the long nightmare of north american chattel slavery. Here Black women were routinely deprived of their breastmilk for the nutritional benefit of white children. This system of biological piracy condemned generations of enslaved Black children to lives of malnutrition while severing their biochemical bonds with their mothers. Ned and Constance Sublette expand on this criminal institution in their 2016 book, *The American Slave Coast: A History of the Slave-Breeding Industry.*

"Enslaved women were used for milk extraction, in the common case of wet nurses, or 'sucklers'—women whose own babies had died or were pushed aside ... Since enslaved women were pregnant so

[3] Perducci, Giulia. "Breastfeeding Animals and Other Wild 'Nurses' in Greek and Roman Mythology." *Gerion*, vol. 34, 2016, pp. 307–323., https://doi.org/10.5209/geri.

[4] Stevens, Emily E, et al. "A History of Infant Feeding." *The Journal of Perinatal Education*, Lamaze International Inc., 2009, https://www.ncbi.nlm.nih.gov/pmc/articles/PMC2684040/.

often, there was little need for a slaveowning white woman to feed her own baby, with the result that baby cotton planters grew up sucking from black women's breasts. Nursing women might be lent out to a family member, or rented out to a stranger. In the latter case, the slaveowner was selling the protein and calcium out of the woman's body.[5]"

Recent studies on the attitudes of Black women on breastfeeding cite this historical trauma as responsible for the negative perceptions some have for this practice. For some Black women, the image of the nursing slave who has no discretion over her milk supply has tainted nursing itself as an activity intrinsically traumatizing and beneath an emancipated people. A more thoughtful response would be to embrace breastfeeding as doing so will enable the Black women of today to provide their children with the psychological and nutritional foundation that their foremothers were cruelly banned from providing. In other words, breastfeeding among Black mothers must be looked upon as **an essential component in maintaining the cultural continuity that we need to thrive as a people.**

Open dialogue about the miseducation and taboos surrounding this most natural of human processes must be put on the community table for examination. The presence of Black fathers in this conversation is mandatory as many of these misperceptions are most pronounced among men. According to a CDC survey analyzing the public opinion of men and women on breastfeeding only 23% of respondents believed breastfeeding could reduce the likelihood of breast cancer and 15% that it could reduce the likelihood of

---

[5] *The American Slave Coast: A History of the Slave-Breeding Industry* – Ned and Constance Sublette (2016)

hypertension and Type 2 diabetes. This is despite easily accessible scientific data attesting to the health benefits of breastfeeding not only in combating cancers and diabetes but also in strengthening overall immunity to infectious diseases and lowering the incidence of postpartum depression

Historically, the source of this mass ignorance about breastfeeding can be traced to the multibillion dollar baby formula industry. In an attempt to displace the mother in pursuit of financial profit, corporations such as Gerber, Similac, and Enfamil infiltrated our homes through mass media advertising. In these highly deceptive exercises in psychological warfare companies pitched these corn-syrup concoctions as the magic cure for mothers struggling to get their baby to latch, experiencing nipple soreness, or just overwhelmed with worry that their newborn wasn't getting enough milk. At a fundamental level this media offensive is about sowing seeds of self-doubt in Black mothers and this self-doubt has since spread like a virus infecting Black fathers, so now we defer to the same corporations compromising on our vow to protect our women in sickness and in health. It is little wonder that breastfeeding among Black women only began to decline and formula substitutes started to take off in the late 1960s and early 1970s, the same period where we were supposed to be celebrating the new day of an "integrated" america. A self-assured, sovereign culture would have been able to discern in this moment that what is "good" for *them* is always lethal for us. When the mothers of our children choose to abandon the power of breastfeeding they are tacitly revealing a lack of trust in their ability to promote life. They are saying that unless they have visual confirmation that nutrients are being supplied (in the form of an emptying baby bottle) they can only nurse their babies uneasily.

The divine force of the Creator dwells in the unseen intersection between the mother's breast and her child. It is this dynamic of feeding, where the baby's biological dependency on the mother stimulates not just a physical but a spiritual transmission, that makes breastfeeding a uniquely empowering act. This spiritual conduit between the mother and child is tragically closed off when formula or bottle feeding is substituted for breastfeeding.

As Black fathers, we must become advocates for neonatal literacy and have the courage to defy mainstream narratives that shame Black mothers or seek to instill fear in them for choosing to nourish our children the natural way. This requires that Black fathers overcome the idea that they are somehow unqualified to give informed counsel about the health of their partners. Yes, mothers have endured three trimesters of gestation and the physical challenges of childbirth and the body is truly intuitive in guiding them towards health and wellness. Yet it is our responsibility to ensure that external actors with ulterior motives do not infringe upon their mental peace by undermining their confidence and assertiveness in this delicate stage of their journey. At the core of the breastfeeding process is a basic self-trust that the mother, with her body alone, is capable of sustaining life. This means she should find easy assurance that her baby is being adequately nourished without having the visual confirmation of a filled bottle (whether it contains pumped breastmilk or formula). The biologically programmed sucking motion of the infant, and the bond this behavior engenders, is sufficient confirmation of health for a self-trusting mother. Beyond the measurable benefits to our children's physical and emotional wellbeing on a social level all functioning institutions and organizations within a culture are formed on the basis that they promote the genetic survival of the members involved. In this sense, breastfeeding not only awakens mothers to their life-giving potential relative to their infant children but, when practiced consistently in a supportive environment, it should activate a broader consciousness of her power as a social agent tasked with the production and stewardship of the people's culture. Refusal to breastfeed by the mother, when she is wholly capable, or the active enabling of this refusal on the part of the father or others is a form of invited collective suicide. **As husbands, we must let the mothers of our children know, without equivocation, that they are fully capable!** Observing the positive health benefits in our son without the use of pumping, but solely breastfeeding through the nipple (responsive feeding), has enhanced the level trust we have in our own sovereign abilities as parents.. Additionally, wise community elders, midwives and doulas, or books such as Dr. Llaila O. Afrika's *African Holistic Health* must be made use of to broaden our literacy so we can be the protectors of life we were born to be.

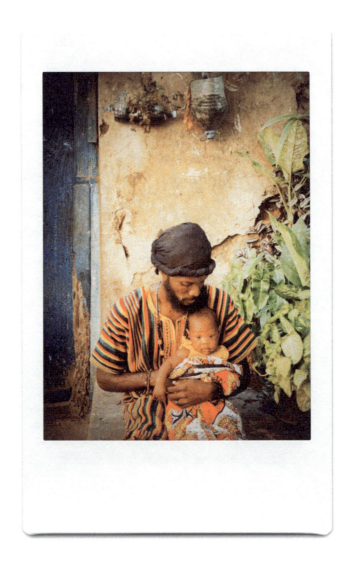

Jahi and I in Bagamoyo, Tanzania

Chapter 2

THE FATHER'S ROLE IN BREASTFEEDING

When we think about the practice of breastfeeding the role of the father is too often overlooked. The bonding between the mother and child is thought to occur without any input from the person who shares half of the baby's DNA. But when we look at breastfeeding from a holistic perspective—one that integrates how the mother child bond factors into the overall family dynamic—the role of the father not only becomes clearer but it is, in all regards, indispensable. When the father is involved in assisting the mother and cultivating a safe environment for feeding the mother is able to successfully transmit the cultural values of the baby, laying the foundation for long-term growth.

"An infant gets subtle acculturation with the rituals and ceremonies of breastfeeding and being with the mother," writes Dr. Llaila O. Afrika in his classic work *African Holistic Health*. "The mother's skin texture, conversations, emotions, behaviors, and movements are ways in which culture is transmitted." It is the father's responsibility to stand guard and ensure this intergenerational transmission takes place. Being attentively present and supplying our women with consistent positive reinforcement can make all the difference between your child benefiting from the biological gift of breastmilk or being faced with the baby formula-induced health difficulties of obesity and constipation. A brief survey of the health benefits of breast milk removes all doubt as to the centrality of breastfeeding as a non-negotiable aspect of neonatal wellness. Health benefits of breastfeeding include:

-Breast Milk is the life-giving waters of the mother

-Baby's saliva communicates with mother's body through the nipple to provide perfect amount of nutrients for the growth and development of the baby

-Transmits culture, body temperature, and emotions from mother to the baby

-Enhances brain chemistry to strengthen the baby's intelligence

-Lays basis for immune system of the baby

-Lays healthy foundation to prevent digestive issues, diarrhea, obesity, and constipation

-Lowers risk of "sudden infant death syndrome" by 36% and lowers risk of ear infections

-Prevents need for speech therapy and strengthens facial muscles

-Passes immune response from mother to child

-Prevents leukemia, diabetes, and hypertension later in life for the baby

-Lower risk for postpartum depression, diabetes, ovarian cancer, and heart disease in mother

According to a 2019-2020 CDC survey only 25.8% of US infants were breastfed exclusively through six months—a global low among "developed" nations—and nearly a fifth (19.4%) of breastfed newborns received, "formula supplementation within the first two days of life."[6] When these figures are weighed alongside the troubling reality that Black mothers are statistically less likely to breastfeed compared to whites, much of it owing to economic pressures of returning to work and inadequate social support systems, Black fathers are obligated to interpret the status quo of Black maternal health as being under a state of siege.

In order to reverse these negative trends there must be a radical reappraisal of our value as fathers and the divine authority we wield in enhancing the lives of our wives and children. This would mean acting on the statistic that husbands who encourage their wives to breastfeed on average breastfeed longer than those husbands who do not. We must begin to encourage co-sleeping as this will structure the environment to be nursing-friendly, lessening the strain of late-night feedings while solidifying the mother-child bond. Community resources in the form of doulas, midwives, and holistic health counselors must be utilized to the fullest to help guide you through the fourth trimester. In addition to facilitating the mental and physical

---

6 Key Breastfeeding Indicators – Centers for Disease Control and Prevention (2021)

challenges that the mother faces, this external intervention will serve as an education for the father to broaden his perspective on the many functions and needs of his partner's anatomy. This must include the development of a menu of food items necessary for adequate milk production. Preparation of these dishes can be done with the assistance of community members or alone but it's essential it be done.

Another aspect of early postpartum care should be the full adoption of around-the-clock breastfeeding as a method of ensuring your baby receives all the nutrients and emotional bonding it needs. This practice, derisively termed "breast feeding on demand" which is better termed "responsive breastfeeding" (a term I like more), is in actuality the most natural and compassionate way to attend to the needs of our babies. Too many families rely on pumping, freezing, and storing breastmilk as an alternative to responsive breastfeeding. It must be understood that closeness and intimacy is the context in which all breastfeeding takes place therefore, bottle feeding your baby breastmilk, while supplying him or her with the necessary nutrients, deprives them of the essential bonding time that can only be experienced through a mother's warmth. Busy job schedules, need for "me-time" (too time consuming), the desire to have other family members participate in feeding, or simply being "touched out," are all cited as justification for rejecting compassionate breastfeeding (breastfeeding on demand). Ignored in this logic is the cultural roots of much of these excuses. For instance, being "touched out" is a relatively new phenomenon that legitimizes the notion that an infant merely expressing its biological dependence upon the mother is somehow a burden. This mentality is borne from a narcissistic, european culture of consumerism that systematically devalues any and everything that does not contribute to personal pleasure or satisfaction. As mature, enlightened parents we must establish the norm that certain practices in regard to the care of our children are to be seen as non-negotiable priorities. Breastfeeding is a non-negotiable priority. When our babies are breastfeed based on their hunger, as opposed to every two hours, we are organizing a schedule based around their needs and not those of the parent. This is an elementary component of imbuing your household with a culture of child-centeredness, which will then contribute greatly to the psychosocial development of your children. Benefits of responsive breastfeeding include: it allows the mother to empty her breasts completely according to the mother and the baby's natural eating cycle, a happier and calmer baby, healthier sleep patterns for the mother and the baby (in the context of co-sleeping), reduces risk of mastitis through regularly draining the breast, the organic creation of a schedule tailored to your baby's needs, establishment of positive relationship with food in the baby's mind as the baby will learn to eat for health instead of hunger (risk factor for obesity), and the promotion of self-regulation in the baby so that he or she never overfeeds, and saves time and money as pumping can be time consuming and expensive. With regard to the self-regulatory effect of responsive breastfeeding when you baby knows when it has had enough milk and stops itself from overconsumption the mother's breast is disciplining the infant on how to have a functional, holistic relationship with food. This carries long term positive consequences in terms of the child psychological and emotional development. If you partner is experiencing difficulty in breastfeeding/lactation consult a lactation specialist who can help assist her in the journey.

All of this should be carried out in the context of taking as much time as possible away from work. We must begin to prioritize the health of our families over any desire for monetary gain. While our role as providers for our families is certainly sacrosanct, we must understand that the most enduring provision that we can supply our families with is bonding time. Any profession that blocks your ability to do this must be reconsidered as a threat to your psychological development. Along with this withdrawal from corporate spaces, we also must psychologically divest from a mainstream white culture defined by the over-sexualizing of women and the fetishizing of breasts. It is this breast fetish culture that is responsible for the territorial attitude some men develop in their failure to encourage the mothers of their children to breastfeed. If the infant is feeding off of the mother's breast whenever it hungers this means nearly all sexual activity involving breasts is indefinitely suspended. This selfish, immature perspective not only devalues your partner's role as a mother but complicates her ability to be confident in feeding her child by making her choose between her newborn and her husband. The constantly evolving "snapback" culture which indoctrinates mothers to believe that having "snatched" abs and an hourglass figure is more important than the nutritional wellbeing of their newborn is an extension of this breast fetish culture that also must be driven from consciousness by all mature, child-centered parents. Finally, we must be determined in purging our home environments of all fear-based negative energy as these are major risk factors in disrupting the spiritual growth of our families during the fourth trimester. Assuming a militant posture when it comes to safeguarding our wives and children in this sensitive period will ensure the creation of functional, lifelong bonds and a breaking of generational traumas that have haunted Black families since the days of slavery. Collectively, as a *true* coalition of men, we can finally put to rest the slanderous image of the disinterested, detached father who prioritizes the empty tokens of white male power over the sacred power of Afrikan fatherhood. Accomplishing that goal begins in the privacy of our own hearts and minds as well as the homes we are sworn to protect.

Chapter 3

FORMULA: IMITATION MILK FOR IMITATION HEALTH

A core feature of all life-centered cultures (Afrikan cultures) is the protection of natural sources of health and sustenance. Whether it be herbal remedies, the healing power of the sun, or the immune boosting breast milk of mothers, nature has more than equipped us to address all health challenges of the body and mind. It is only with the rapid rise of western industrial society and its unrestrained appetite for profit that this holistic paradigm of growth and development has been shattered.

In the realm of maternal care the obscenely lucrative baby formula industry fills this role. According to a recent report in *GlobeNewswire*, the baby formula market is expected to grow at an annual rate of 9.8% and, "is anticipated to reach around USD 110.26 billion by 2026." The detrimental health consequences of formula "milk" are well documented and must be considered by all Black fathers who are intent on providing their children with the adequate nutrition for balanced living.

Harmful health effects and deficiencies of formula "milk" include:

-The inability to provide the baby with immune boosting antibodies needed to fight infections. **"None of the antibodies found in breast milk are manufactured in formula."**

-Doesn't adapt its chemical composition to meet the nutritional needs of the baby

-Increases digestive issues such as constipation and gas.

-Produces firmer and harder stool (bowel movements).

-Increase likelihood of eczema, asthma, and food allergies in infant (Atopy)

Central to the propaganda of the baby formula industry is the notion that this manufactured, lab-made product is a legitimate competitor with breastmilk or can be considered "milk" at all. Formula must be understood as a dangerous imitation milk. Imitation milk, "has indigestible artery-clogging saturated hydrogenated coconut oil, excess estrogen, steroids, growth hormones, sodium caseinate from milk or soybeans, corn syrup (white sugar product), salt, emulsifiers, dyes, potassium phosphate, artificial flavors and acidic synthetic vitamins and minerals."[7] As a finished product, this chemical concoction functions as a gateway drug to unhealthy eating habits which normalizes obesity, constipation, and excess waste as desirable.

When hugely influential formula corporations like Nestle or Abbott advocate that Black mothers mix formula with breastmilk— what industry reps deceptively call "supplementing"—they are purposely concealing the known fact that the less a baby suckles the nipple of his or her mother the *less* the mother will lactate. Instead of calling this process "supplementing" it should be called what it actually is: *weaning the mother off of her own breast milk*.

More disturbingly, the force of this corporate attack is aided by a mass media culture more interested in generating ad revenue than being a genuine check on power. In a *VeryWellFamily* article headlined, "Combining Breastfeeding and Formula Feeding," Donna Murray, RN, writes that it's "perfectly safe" for mothers to resort to formula feeding. Among the reasons listed for supplementing breast milk with formula is if the mother is, "going back to work", "your partner wants to participate", "you have multiples" (more than one baby), "you have low breast milk supply", "your child has medical issues", or—shockingly— "you just want to." To make matters worse this health "advice" was given within an illustration of a Black mother (with no father in sight) reaching into a mini refrigerator stocked full of imitation milk.

Overcoming this misinformation requires an outgrowing of selfish tendencies that place the personal satisfaction of the mother

---

[7] *African Holistic Health* [Revised and Expanded 7th Edition] – Dr. Llaila O. Afrika (2009)

above the mutually beneficial mother-child relationship and its central role in the overall health of the family. As Black fathers, we are uniquely positioned to construct a solid wall of defense against these corporate entities intent on breaking apart this most sacred of biochemical bonds. It is the mother's breast which bonds the child to the culture of its people and its ancestors. Conversely, baby formula bonds your child to the culture of the formula manufacturers (white culture) and the governmental agencies that provide them safe haven to launch their attacks. Considering the fact that there is no verifiable health benefit attached to formula feeding, it is apparent that the problem we face is wholly psychological in nature. Like so much else in the cultural agenda to demonize Black motherhood, the diminishment of the confidence of the mother as it relates to her ability to provide for the nutritional needs for her baby is key to preserving the status quo. Only a conscientious uprising of Black fathers can help mend this psychological void to heal our families. Practical measures that Black fathers can adopt to encourage exclusive breastfeeding include:

‑Mastering methods to soothe your baby when he or she cries as the baby's cry may increase distress and worry in mothers with lactation challenges. Any experience of a delay or scarcity in milk production may lead them to believe a "quick fix" is needed in the form of formula as opposed to patiently waiting for their body to respond to meet the baby's needs. (See Chapter on Father Bonding Techniques)

‑Educating yourself and your partner on the deceptive marketing and linguistic tricks that formula corporations use to convince mothers that they are inadequate.

-Purging your household of all baby formula products, literature, and paraphernalia. Hospitals give out formula free as a bait for mothers to discontinue breastfeeding. We must value our role as protectors by ensuring these corrupt influences do not intrude upon our homes. (See Chapter on Protecting the Perimeter).

-Providing genuine, consistent, and enthusiastic praise and encouragement to your partner as she passes breastfeeding milestones (3 months, 6 months, 1 year, etc.) Breastfeeding is not only beneficial to the mother and the child but to fathers as well. It anchors the mother and the child in their culture and makes it easier for fathers to communicate with them both without the conflicting interests that characterize dysfunctional white families (See Oedipus Complex).

It is also critical that we not compare the temperament of our breastfed babies with the temperament of formula fed babies. Studies have conclusively shown that breastfed babies on average cry more, sleep less, and are more active. These traits often dissuade parents from breastfeeding because they interpret this higher level of energy or irritability as a problem. Instead these behaviors are completely natural and represent a complex system of signaling whereby the baby is communicating its nutritional needs to the mother. When babies are bottle fed formula milk the parent is socializing them to eat for comfort (comfort eating) instead of eating for nutrition. Furthermore, "research suggests that these [formula fed] infants may be over-nourished and gain weight too quickly." So, while parents may be getting more rest from their seemingly more content and "happy" babies fed on formula this happiness is attained at the price of their baby's long term health. Do not equate a "happy" baby with a healthy baby.

Bottle Feeding Breastmilk is Not Breastfeeding

Breaking free of the misinformation that says a "happy" baby is a healthy baby will also require mothers disown the notion that feeding their babies breastmilk via a bottle is no different than feeding them through the nipple. Breastfeeding through the nipple has specific emotional, psychological, and spiritual benefits which are lost in transmission during bottle feeding. One of the primary ways breastfeeding through the nipple differs from bottle feeding deals with the transfer of the mother's temperature to the infant via her breast milk. In the transfer of the mother's temperature via breast milk there is a corresponding transfer of the mother's temperament —her mood, attitudes, emotions, and general demeanor. When mothers withhold, or replace the nipple with the artificial nipple of the baby bottle they are effectively de-spiritualizing the process of breastfeeding and creating a space for bond damage to occur. Because while the baby is identifying his or her mother as the supreme source of life when receiving its nutritional intake through the mother's nipple it identifies the bottle as that source when bottle fed. Later in life this misidentification comes through in the child's materialistic attachments to physical objects at the expense of more meaningful, non-material spiritual relationships. Freezing breastmilk for storage to be used for later feeding is also a way to further disrupt and de-spiritualize the breastfeeding process. A baby that is consuming breastmilk whose temperature has been radically altered through freezing, refrigeration, or boiling is bound to become estranged from the temperament of the mother because the very substance that was designed to instill that temperament has been manipulated beyond recognition. Scientific research aligns with this critique of bottle feeding underscoring not only its shortcomings in comparison to breastfeeding but also its inherent risk factors. Risk factors of bottle feeding include[8]:

- Interference with the comfort, closeness, soothing effect, and security that comes with breastfeeding (See M.T.C.)
- Dis-regulates eating habits, creating a precursor for eating disorders
- Increase probability of coughing and wheezing in infant
- Freezing breast milk compromises its immunological benefits
  - Freezing breast milk reduces its antioxidant properties
  - Microwaving breast milk decreases its anti-infective properties
  - Increased probability of baby only consuming "hind milk" (high in carbohydrates)
  - Increased probability of bacterial infection via contaminated bottles
  - Disrupts the suck/swallow/breathe cycle

When a mother is breastfeeding her child, she is instilling within that child its very first concept of God as a divine sustainer. A child

---

[8] Campbell, Olivia. The Unseen Consequences of Pumping Breast Milk. *Pacific Standard*, Pacific Standard, 17 Nov. 2014, https://psmag.com/economics/unseen-consequences-pumping-breast-milk-94181.

who has a mother who practices responsive breastfeeding (See Chapter 2)—feeding the child according to the child's emotional and nutritional needs—will cultivate a concept of God within her child that is loving and protective. Conversely, a mother who bottle feeds her child (depriving that child of the nipple and the biochemical benefits attached to it) will likewise cultivate a concept of God in her child that is selfish and neglectful. Breastmilk is a living substance and like every other living organism on earth it operates within a strictly designed life cycle. When the crucial transfer milk from the nipple of the mother to the mouth of the child is bypassed it unnecessarily interrupts that life cycle which is kept active through the saliva of the baby interacting with the skin of the mother. The reciprocity that is the foundation stone of all balanced relationships is broken and the baby is unable to reflect back to the mother the positive energies that she imparts to him or her.

When we sincerely invest in these productive ways of thinking and patterns of behavior we are nurturing a revolutionary, subversive culture in our homes that is able to withstand the most determined of foes. Breast Milk directly from the nipple is the chemical foundation of that culture that no bottle could ever replace.

<u>Comparing Feeding Cycles</u>

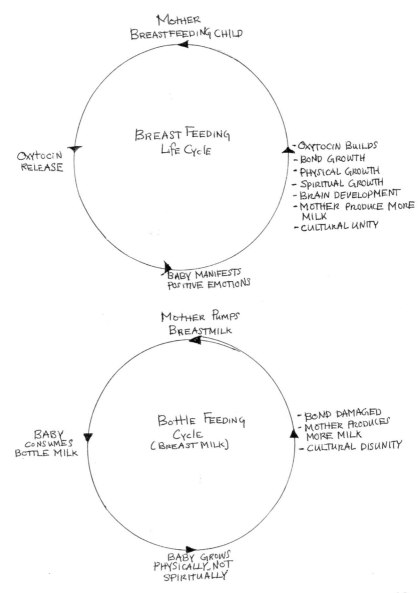

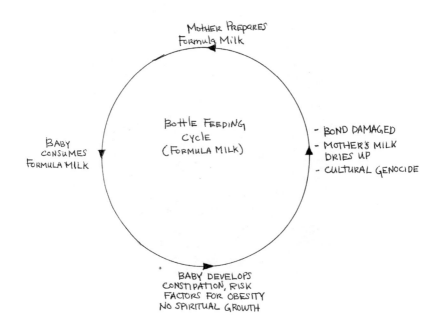

MOTHER PREPARES
Formula Milk

BOTTLE FEEDING
CYCLE
(FORMULA MILK)

BABY
CONSUMES
FORMULA MILK

- BOND DAMAGED
- MOTHER'S MILK
  DRIES UP
- CULTURAL GENOCIDE

BABY DEVELOPS
CONSTIPATION, RISK
FACTORS FOR OBESITY
NO SPIRITUAL GROWTH

41

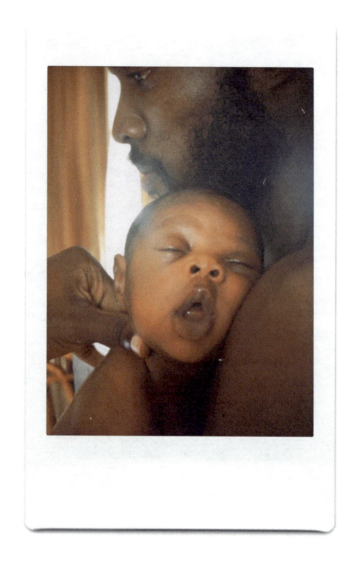

Soothing Jahi to sleep via skin-to-skin

Chapter 4

FATHER'S ROLE IN PREVENTING EARLY PAIN AND TRAUMA IN OUR BABIES

Hospital birth is an initiation into techniques of medicalized torture. This may seem like an extreme statement to some but it highlights a disturbing truth upon closer analysis. In the English dictionary torture is variously defined as, "unbearable physical pain", "extreme mental distress", or "the act of distorting something so it seems to mean something it was not intended to mean." On all counts the highly mechanized and de-spiritualized procedures of child birthing carried out in western hospitals fit this description.

Psychologist and hypnotherapist David Chamberlain criticized this trauma based birthing culture through his work examining patients who were able to recollect their own birth experiences and even prenatal life within the womb. His research also concluded that infants were able to demonstrate signs of consciousness in utero at twenty weeks and could also recognize the voice of the mother in utero at twenty-five weeks (before brain development was complete). These findings refuted decades of medical practice that operated under the assumption that newborns have a deficiency of brain matter and therefore cannot feel pain. Not only are newborns highly sensitive to the painful procedures that hospital staff inflict upon them at birth but the psychological imprint of these traumatic interventions follow them into early childhood, adolescence, and adulthood. As a result, medical professionals in the west are emotionally and psychologically crippling our children with the silent, uninformed consent of Black parents. The following procedures comprise a brief sample of some of the violent methods of birthing endorsed by western hospitals.

PREMATURE CUTTING OF THE UMBILICAL CORD

Second to the mother's breast, in the unfolding of neonatal life no organ is as critical to laying the basis for nutritional wellness than the placenta. Attached to the newborn via a pulsating umbilical cord, this figurative "tree of life" supplies vital nutrients and oxygen to the developing fetus, regulating the baby's breathing patterns and sense of wholeness. When medical teams prematurely cut the umbilical cord, they are not only shutting down this nutrient intake but violently disrupting the rhythmic cycle of the baby's breath. Once this breathing cycle is altered it can never be restored; hence the premature cutting of the umbilical cord should be looked upon as inflicting irreversible damage to the emotional and psychological potential of a baby. From a biological perspective, it is the control of the breath that is at the center of balanced living. How are we to raise our children to be models of order and balance (Maat) if the precondition for this is terminated at birth? (For more on this see chapter on Placenta Birth).

SEPARATION FROM MOTHER AND DELAYING SKIN-TO-SKIN

In the critical first seconds after the birth of our baby it is imperative that the baby and its mother establish skin-to-skin contact. This facilitates the release of the chemical called oxytocin which aids in the cognitive and emotional bonding of the mother and child. Tragically, this essential task is completely ignored in western hospitals. Instead newborns are swiftly taken away from their mothers to cold rooms where they are placed in incubators under bright, fluorescent lights. The psychological pain endured by the infant, newly released from the biochemical security of its mother's womb to be thrust into an alien environment full of white coats, white masks, white lights, and white people must register in the brains of Black infants as a traumatic event approximating death. We must understand that when we enter hospitals we are metaphorically putting our children in white hands as a preparation for doing this literally. When the psychological costs of this transfer of authority is weighed, we should understand that one second in their hands is one second too many.

UNNECESSARY C-SECTIONS

Caesarian sections (C-sections) are increasingly becoming the procedure of choice for western hospitals, almost always at the expense of the health of the mother and child. Nearly a third of all hospital births in america (31%) are conducted via C-section with Black women being the largest demographic subjected to this surgical procedure (35%). The rationale given for carrying out C-sections by hospital workers often include mental coercion in the form of instilling fear ("unless you get a C-section your baby might die") and fallacious reasoning such as the notion that a mother who gave birth via C-section for her first child must, for her own "safety", also give birth this way for all subsequent children. Enforcement of this reckless, deceptive policy is a key contributor to the escalating maternal mortality rates among Black women, with a large portion of these hospital deaths being attributed to C-section related complications like infections, sepsis, and post-natal hemorrhaging. According to Dr. Llaila O. Afrika, "C section babies have an increase in diseases, bonding difficulties and learning problems." Other adverse health outcomes associated with C-Sections include:

- Autoimmune disorders
- Asthma
- Type II Diabetes
- Obesity
- Gastrointestinal, Respiratory, and Viral Infections

On a historical note, the origin of the word "Caesarian" is a decree authored by Caesar in the Roman legal code which mandated that, "all women who were so fated by childbirth must be cut open." The sole application of this decree was in "post-mortem operations"—the accepted norm being that C-sections were reserved exclusively for mothers who were either dead or dying. "Above all it was a measure of last resort, and **the operation was not intended to preserve the mother's life.**" Occasionally, a live fetus would be extracted from the womb of a dead mother so as to contribute to the empire's population numbers. This savage tradition continued without serious alteration until the 19th century where it was incorporated into western "science" as a legitimate feature of "medical education."[9] Other perversions which underlie the white resort to C-sections is the desire to preserve the vagina of the mother for the sexual pleasure of the man or what they obscenely label the

---

[9] "Caesarean Section – A Brief History", US National Library of Medicine (National Institute of Health, 2013).

"honeymoon vagina."[10] The "honeymoon vagina" is borne from a patriarchal culture of white male domination that seeks to deny the life-giving potential of the female anatomy in service of their sexual appetites. From this phobia surrounding the vagina emerges a vocabulary of phrases (comparison of vagina to flowers and cherries, etc.) and socially trained squeamishness when it comes to examining the particulars of vaginal birth. This reveals how western medical practice cannot be separated from western culture and how we as a people descended from an Afrikan culture have no business entrusting our women or children to their "care."

INDUCING BIRTH OR INDUCING DISTRESS?

One of the more distinct features of the assembly line model of birthing practiced by western medical institutions is the over-reliance on induced births as a so-called "safety" measure for Black mothers. Stimulated by the use of Pitocin—**a drug often administered without the signed consent of mothers**—these induced births are the primary causes of fetal distress and form the rationale for many C-Sections. After receiving a dose of Pitocin, the baby, in a panicked state, defecates in the womb (meconium). This

10 Mathur, Vani A., et al. "Cultural Conceptions of Women's Labor Pain and Labor Pain Management: A Mixed-Method Analysis." *Social Science & Medicine*, Pergamon, 27 July 2020, https://www.sciencedirect.com/science/article/pii/S0277953620304597#bib65.

prenatal bowel movement not only contaminates the placenta but makes necessary its immediate extraction from the womb so as to prevent the fetus from ingesting fecal bacteria. Arguments for inducing birth often follow the usage of fetal baby monitors, an instrument which is known to produce distress in unborn infants. This distress is then used as a pretext to induce birth while ignoring that the doctors created the distress in the first place. Sane medical practice will allow the mother's body to naturally birth the baby without interfering with the balance of hormonal chemicals needed for proper bonding. In western hospital settings inducing birth is code for inducing fetal and maternal distress.

CIRCUMCISION

A number of baby boys die each year due to hospital administered circumcisions. These incisions removing the foreskin from the genitals of newborns defies any sound medical logic. The culture of circumcision in western cultures centers around the perverse need to control the sexual development of dominated peoples. Just as young girls, in some cultures, have their clitoris removed to numb sexual sensations later in life so too does male circumcision come out of this background of european psychosexual disorder. Furthermore, hospitals routinely use the foreskin cut from the penises of newborns for stem cell medical research (much like the placentas extracted from birthing mothers). *Discover* magazine gives a nod to this practice in an article disturbingly headlined, "Why Human Foreskin is a Hot

Commodity in Science," where reporter Molly Glick hails the benefits of human foreskin in, "testing revolutionary drugs," and "repairing human organs."[11] That the cost of acquiring this "hot commodity" is strapping newborns to operating tables to be casually mutilated while they scream in agony is considered too trivial to mention. As stated at the outset of this chapter, newborns are acutely aware of their environment and possess the consciousness and sensory ability to register pain just as much as anyone else. When parents voluntarily subject their children to these procedures they are ignorantly doing so under the assumption that the baby doesn't feel pain. This is false and a tacit endorsement of medical torture. Long-term negative health outcomes of circumcision include erectile dysfunction, difficulty achieving orgasm, and premature ejaculation. When socialized into a mainstream media culture fixated on consumerism and sexual pleasure circumcised males make ideal candidates for sexually dysfunctional beings unable to transcend the appetite driven regions of their lower selves.

Phrases all Black fathers should look out for if forced to engage with western medical institutions include:
1. "Your baby is too big"
2. "Your baby's heart rate is dropping"
3. "If the baby doesn't come out soon we'll have to do a C-section"
4. "Not cutting the cord is useless."

---

[11] "Why Human Foreskin is a Hot Commodity in Science"- Glick, Molly. *Discover*. July, 26, 2021.

5. "Since your first birth was a C-section, vaginal birth is too dangerous."

6. "Breech births must be delivered via C-section to protect you and the baby."

7. "We have to administer vaccines to protect the public."

8. "Babies don't feel pain."

If any of these phrases are used in your presence it is imperative you intervene and advocate on behalf of your wife. **If doctors persist this is medical coercion and you must leave the area immediately.**

Apart from these tactics of linguistic manipulation, the health status of Black mothers is often cited as a reason to resort to these violently invasive methods (induction of birth, C-Sections, cutting of umbilical cord and disposal of placenta). Preeclampsia or hypertension is one of the most widespread risk factors that afflict Black mothers in america. This epidemic of high blood pressure is traceable to low-nutrition diets devoid of whole foods rich in vital minerals and fiber. Studies show that Black women are "far more likely to have preeclampsia than white women" (60% greater chance). While 70 out of 1,000 Black women were diagnosed with preeclampsia only 43 out 1,000 white women were diagnosed. Of the white women diagnosed cases were described as "mild." More revealingly, Black women born in america have a "higher risk of developing high blood pressure ... compared to black women who immigrated to the country." Black women who immigrated to america had a 27% lower risk of having preeclampsia than american born Black women and the risk of immigrant Black women getting preeclampsia increased, "after they lived in the US for more than 10 years." What this data suggests is that the high incidence of hypertension among pregnant Black women is a biological trademark of living in a society organized around the destruction of Black motherhood. This should motivate us as Black fathers to support our life partners during pregnancy to adopt a natural whole foods diet for the family (husband and wife). In addition to warding off the maternal health complications associated with high blood pressure such a change in eating habits would help to cultivate growth-based bonds within our marriages where our health, the health of our wives, and the health of our unborn are intimately linked. The de-spiritualization of the birthing process can only be defeated once we take the responsibility to re-spiritualize our homes. Transforming how we think and act vis-à-vis the larger mainstream white society is integral to this process.

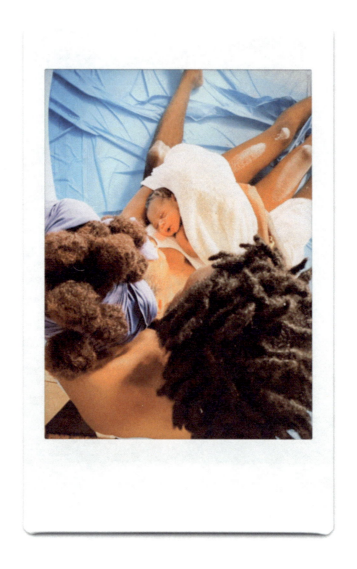

In the birthing pool moments after Jahi's arrival

Chapter 5

HOME BIRTH: WHERE THE REVOLUTIONARY FATHER IS BORN

"The unborn child takes the man and woman on an emotional journey (Rites of Passage). The unborn child causes the man and woman's feelings and emotions to touch the unborn child inside themselves. The unborn child is birthing the man and woman as a mother and father (parents)."
-Dr. Llaila O. Afrika

I awakened to my wife pacing across the room, talking on the phone in a lowered tone. She was at 38 weeks and I knew the birth of our first child together was imminent. As our doula, Osun

Wunmi[12], calling in from the states, coached her through the contractions I headed downstairs to the living room to fill the birthing pool with water. It was a little past 4am, the sun had yet to peek over the horizon but the roosters were crowing in excited anticipation. After emptying the twenty or so 12 liter jugs into the pool and pulling the water hose through the back window to complete the process, the space for the birth of our child was ready. By this point my wife's water had broken and her medicine ball provided the only relief from the many contractions which racked her body with intense frequency. Time was of the essence and I had to get her to the pool down stairs. Everything was happening so fast. My body was moving, as if by reflex, ahead of all doubt with urgent deliberateness. There was no fatigue, nervousness, worry, or uncertainty. All of my energy was singularly focused on ensuring a safe passage for my unborn child. Nothing else, at that moment, mattered.

Once downstairs, my wife continued doing hip-rolls on the medicine ball while I alternated between warming up the pool with heated water and applying double-hip squeezes to her lower back to help the labor progress more smoothly. The woman's body knows instinctively what it needs, when it needs it, and how to satisfy that need. Watching my wife vocalize her needs without hesitation to me and our doula underscored how critical the mother's independent voice is when conducting a safe, healthy, trauma free birth. "We're having a baby." She said this mid-hip roll while smiling. It was at that point that I truly understood the psychological significance of my

---

[12] Osun Wunmi is a licensed doula who operates virtually and physically through her Prestigious Doula Academy organization.

supportive presence. Though she was enduring the sacrificial pain of labor it was indeed *we* who was birthing our child. The hour was approaching 7am, my son Mikey had awakened and was assisting me in warming up the water. He too evidenced no fear, nervousness, or uncertainty. The family dynamic was organized to achieve the goal of safeguarding life.

"I feel like I need to push. I need to get in the water." The contractions were finally approaching its climatic end as I helped her into the pool. "Baba, the kettle is smoking," said Mikey. I ran to the kitchen to find the kettle in flames. Quickly unplugging it and rushing to the backyard to put the fire out my wife yells from the living room. "The head is out!" I throw the smoldering kettle into the grass and dash back into the living room. Our baby's head is out completely! I lower myself into the water behind my wife, caressing her leg, awaiting that final contraction. In one swift motion, as if by propulsion, our baby wholly emerges in the water. My wife lifts him out and rests his body on her left breast, establishing skin-to-skin contact and initiating the sacred bond at the root of all healthy psychological development. In three short hours, I had delivered my son without the "aid" of epidurals, Pitocin, forceps, fetal baby monitors, white medical doctrines, or white physicians. We had a successful birth relying exclusively on our community, our knowledge, our study, our belief in ourselves and our Creator. In delivering my son into this life I was able to deliver myself and my family into another life, a life where fear is just a figment of the abused mind and health is the ability to act conscientiously on behalf of your people's self-preservation. As Black fathers, we come into a greater understanding of our role as protectors and guardians of life by fully investing ourselves in the birthing process. On November 19,

2021, I experienced what revolutionary power feels like. This is the spiritual gift of homebirth.

BRIEF HISTORICAL BACKGROUND ON HOMEBIRTHS

For the majority of our history home birth has been the cultural standard for Black people. Whether we are speaking of the varied birthing rituals from continental Africa or the plantation midwives during our captivity in north america, we have always relied upon the wisdom of our elders and resources within our community to usher new life into this world. In the slave south, where midwives, were recognized as the cultural authorities in matters of childbirth Black women relied upon the doctrine of "Motherwit," to ensure safe passage of the unborn. Writing on the history of Black midwifery in the 20th century South author Jenny Luke describes Motherwit as, "a blend of God-given wisdom and common sense that was usually in the possession of older women."[13] This commonsensical approach to birthing was built upon an identity of values between the midwife and the mother-to-be which distrusted the "scientific" theories of white physicians though they often intervened in the birth rituals of

---

[13] Luke, Jenny M. Delivered by Midwives: African American Midwifery in the Twentieth-Century   South. University Press of Mississippi, 2018.

Black mothers to deadly effect. During slavery, it was not uncommon for expectant mothers to shield their pregnancies from white physicians out of justified fear that their interventions would lead to their deaths or the deaths of their babies.

Following emancipation and the so-called modernization of healthcare at the turn of the century clinics and hospitals began to replace the traditional home birth environments of Black mothers. But the advances in technology did little to alleviate maternal mortality in the Deep South. An estimated 1 in 25 C-sections performed on Black mothers in 1939 Alabama resulted in death and of all the systematically underfunded clinics—a "colored institution"—of Alabama not a single one had a labor ward. This was typical in a nation constructed upon the psychopathic agenda of exploiting Black mothers as slave "breeding" units akin to cows, chickens, hogs, and horses—what historians Ned and Constance Sublette refer to as the "capitalized womb." In Sunflower County Mississippi 60% of Black women who entrusted the birth of their children to white physicians were secretly given postpartum hysterectomies. Horror stories such as this should be at the front of our minds when Black mothers of today enter white hospitals with the expectation of humane treatment.[14]

As the medical abuse of the early 20th century continued apace after the Second World War new policies were introduced to further assimilate Black women into the mainstream medical system. The legal foundation of this social engineering was the Emergency Maternal and Infant Care Program. Spearheaded by the US Children's

---

[14] CNN reports that Black babies are three times more likely to die when in the "care" of white physicians than white babies.

Bureau this legislation sought to propagandize Black women that the midwives which they had been relying on for so long were truly uneducated, un-scientific, laypersons engaged in medical malpractice and the best solution for Black mothers was to opt for the westernized hospital system. Though there was zero evidence to suggest whites were trustworthy candidates to oversee the delivery of our children the deceptive promise of social equality overwhelmed all common sense. By 1969 90% of Black mothers in South Carolina had hospital births, a huge departure from the thinking twenty years earlier when 60% of Black women had midwife managed home births. This organized campaign to eliminate the midwife as a legitimate factor in Black birth culture was completed in 1960 with the passage of Medicaid which allocated state monies to cover the medical costs of expectant mothers while excluding any coverage for midwives. Doulas, the more recent addition to non-hospitalized birth culture, are also excluded from Medicaid coverage.

THE POWER OF PHYSIOLOGIC BIRTH (NATURAL BIRTH)

Physiologic births are natural, vaginal births which are qualitatively superior to hospital births because they prioritize the discretion of the mother in dictating the birth process and the environment in which she gives birth. Trusting the maternal instincts of the mother over the male-centric doctrines of white physicians is at the core of the physiologic birth process. From a natural perspective, the labor process is biologically compelled to shut down when the mother is in an unsafe birthing environment. "A hospital can be the worst place to be for a healthy woman in early labor," according to natural birth website SpiritualBirth.net. Hospitals are, "full of worried people, rules and deadlines, bright lights and clinical technology—all items that will shut down a woman's natural body functions and cause her labor to cease." This explains why inducing labor is such a common practice in hospitals—the natural maternal instinct to delay labor in unsafe environments has to be forcibly bypassed.

Verified benefits of natural home birth for mothers include:

-Higher likelihood of breastfeeding
-Reduced chance of postpartum surgery
-More involved decision making and support
-Reduced cost and less likely to experience C-section

Verified benefits for infants include:

-Reduced likelihood of fetal distress associated with hospital birth
-Reduced likelihood of chronic disease from C-section and delayed breastfeeding
-Improved mother-child bonding

Studies also show that mothers who experience complications while in a home birth setting still have positive birth outcomes without the intervention of a hospital physician. Much of this is traceable to the innate advantages of vaginal birth which, unlike hospital administered C-sections, provides the fetus with microbiota for digestive health and the bonding chemical of oxytocin while lowering the risk of childhood and adult disease.

We must value homebirth and the natural birthing processes that it enshrines because controlling the physical and mental environment during labor helps to lay the foundation for our child's psychological and emotional wellness. The mothers of our children value our presence and when we are next to them they are reminded that they are not on this journey alone. As Black fathers, we are sincerely committing to the mothers of our children by providing the spiritual and moral support they need to transcend the physical pain of childbirth. Birth sovereignty at its core is about more than choosing the techniques of labor but, more importantly, the ambience in which this rite of passage takes place. By doing this we can insulate the women in our lives from invasive, unsolicited influences so that she can birth our children on her own terms.

Practical steps mothers can take to ensure a safe and healthy home birth include:

-Maintaining a positive outlook in regard to the physical and psychological challenges associated with natural home birth. Speak life-affirming statements over yourself such as, "my birth is divine", "my body is designed for life", "my labor will be safe, short, and successful", and "everything I need is within me"

-Only watch non-traumatic home births online. Part of mentally preparing for home birth is knowing millions of women have had successful home births free of trauma and complications. This means refrain from watching any birth videos where women are screaming in agony.

-Trust and be gentle with yourself as you experience the physiological transformations (morning sickness, back pain, mood swings, etc.) of pregnancy. This is all a natural part of the life-giving process and you have the mental resolve to push through it.

-Make regular use of medicine ball. This helps with the proper positioning of the baby's head and will also make for faster labor. The medicine ball is beneficial for both the pregnancy period and during labor.

-Drink plenty of okra water. It has many dietary benefits for pregnant mothers but it also facilitates the labor process by enabling the baby to slip out the womb much easier due to the slimy texture of the vegetable.

-Eat dates throughout the third trimester of your pregnancy. Incorporating dates into your diet will shorten your labor time because it softens the cervix.

-After 37 weeks into your pregnancy drink red raspberry tea. This tea will lessen the pain associated with uterine contractions while also shortening your labor.

-Consult with your doula to help alleviate any fears and also check with your doula to make sure you aforementioned steps are appropriate for your particular pregnancy.

THE BIOPSYCHOSOCIAL FACTORS OF LABOR PAIN

As someone who has witnessed two natural homebirths firsthand, I better understand that reclaiming our power over the birthing process calls for a holistic redefinition of pain and its role in child labor. In both home births I witnessed neither was characterized by expressions of extreme pain. This was entirely due to the fact that homebirth addresses the intricacies of how pain is generated and how best to contain it. Despite these experiences attesting to the safety and security of home birth, mainstream media portrayals of child birth highlight excruciating pain as its defining feature. This has been major deterrent for many Black mothers who may be considering home birth. Hollywood movies depicting mothers (largely white) screaming at the top of their lungs, swearing, and begging for an epidural has completely corrupted our perception of child birth as a burden to be endured instead of a sacred rite to be celebrated. Added to this media propaganda is a theological description of labor pain as God's punishment to women for the "original sin" of eating from the tree of knowledge. This dogma flies in the face of more ancient traditions in North Afrika and Mycenae where Afrikan fertility clans called Sibyls honored child labor as a spiritual achievement integral to the advancement of the matriarchal culture of "mother-right." As Black parents, we must understand that western portrayals of child labor negate the true essence of labor pain as the final product of a series of interactions between the mother's biological and psychological state, and the society in which she is birthing or what the journal of *Social Science and Medicine* calls the, "biopsychosocial nature of pain." Pain during child birth is not exclusively the result of the physiological changes taking place in the mother's body. Of equal importance is the psychological perspective she brings to the process (is laboring a welcome sacrifice or an unwanted burden) and whether or not the social environment she is in reinforces positive, life-affirming behaviors or negative, fear based behavior. When we choose home birth as the only way to bring our children into the world we are prioritizing the multidimensional nature of labor pain and better positioning ourselves to control this pain through the control of the social setting we are in and thoughts we allow to take root. By choosing homebirth the mother, father, and trusted birth workers set the pain threshold whereas in hospital settings this is set by majority white medical teams.

Navigating this complex maze of influences to arrive at some fundamental truth about labor pain will first require an analysis of western cultural messaging and behaviors that limit the agency of Black mothers. One of the primary ways western hospitals induce pain is by the instilling of fear. Studies have shown that the release of oxytocin during child birth acts as a natural painkiller but when the mother is made to feel fearful—a common occurrence in the highly-mechanized methods of hospital delivery—the flow of this spiritually potent chemical is interrupted or as a recent paper researching this topic states:

"The affective component of labor pain also relates to the positive feedback loop ... involving the body's production of oxytocin, which produces labor contractions. **Fear can disrupt this loop, causing labor to stall or contractions to be more painful.**"

Another study on the same topic, but from the perspective of how social factors influence pain, states: "... a determining factor of a woman's experience of pain during labour is **the meaning she ascribes to it.** When women interpret the pain as **productive and purposeful, it is associated with positive cognitions and** emotions, and they are more likely to feel they can cope. Alternatively, when women interpret the pain as threatening, it is associated with **negative cognitions and emotions and they tend to feel they need help from external methods of pain control.**"[15] Apart from this general neglect on the part of mainstream medicine of the social factors that influence how mothers experience pain, is a western cultural fixation on the vagina itself as the sole source of pain and not an interaction between their bodies and the broader psychological/social events unfolding within or around them during child labor. This "overwhelming focus on the sensory definition of pain," is the principal reason why a large majority (87%) of respondents in a 2020 study on labor pain reported that labor pain should be treated medically while a small minority (13%) reported that it should not. In the same study 32% of respondents reported that there is "no value" in labor pain, which is undoubtedly a leading motive in the resort to the use of epidurals. Ultimately, in an attempt to combat this general aversion to pain the report concluded that, **"valuing the pain of labor may provide a perspective that diminishes the desire to ameliorate the pain,"** and **"conceptualizing labor pain as purposeful and productive may decrease the subjective experience of one's labor pain."** Simply put, Black mothers make themselves more susceptible to negative experiences of labor pain when there exists an ignorance about the

15 Whitburn, Laura Y., et al. The Meaning of Labour Pain: How the Social Environment and Other Contextual Factors Shape Women's Experiences - BMC Pregnancy and Childbirth. *BioMed Central*, BioMed Central, 30 May 2017, https://bmcpregnancychildbirth.biomedcentral.com/articles/10.1186/s12884-017-1343-3.Â

biopsychosocial nature of pain and, by the same token, they equip themselves to better manage these experiences when they are properly informed so that they can fashion environments in line with this understanding.

In other areas of the social domain, the white liberal glorification of "equality" as the political remedy for all dysfunctions within the Black community has misled many Black mothers to seek access to epidurals as a solution to deal with the pain of child labor. Statistics show that Black women on average use epidurals less than white women (even those white women who are uninsured) and much of this is due to the western belief that Black people, by their nature, feel less pain than whites. Disregarding what the white medical establishment says, we should be making decisions based on the cultural practices of our ancestors, not in reaction to the legal and cultural norms of a race of people who have never held the maternal health of Black mothers in high regard (with or without epidurals). The genetic and cultural origins of white women compel them to use artificial aids such as epidurals, Pitocin, and C-sections in the laboring process because, unlike Black women, they lack the anatomy to easily accommodate the physical challenges of natural labor. Our ancestors were not only child-centered but through a finely tuned system of spiritual practice and ritual were able to organize their social environments and raise their psychological state to such a level that labor pain was not avoided but embraced head on. As strong, self-determined Black fathers, we should be encouraging the mothers of our children to participate in this tradition through unmedicated, natural homebirth. Holistic ways to help manage the pain of childbirth include the consuming of okra water, only speaking positive affirmations, only consuming media that displays women birthing in peaceful, serene, and life-affirming environments, steering clear of "birth horror stories", smiling through contractions, focusing on pain as integral to the labor process and not an interference or signal that something is wrong, and avoiding people/environments that are motivated by fear. Below is a partial list of positive confessions that can be spoken prior to and during child labor that my wife and I created:

1. **My labor is going to be short**

2. **I honor my ancestors when I birth naturally**

3. **My contractions draw me closer to my baby**

4. **I trust everyone around me**

5. **There is beauty in sacrifice**

6. **Birthing and breastfeeding is healing for my mind, body, and spirit**

7. **I have the power to feed nations through my breast**

8. **Contractions bond me with my baby**

9. **My baby is healthy, whole, and complete**

10. **Childbirth brings me closer to my Creator**

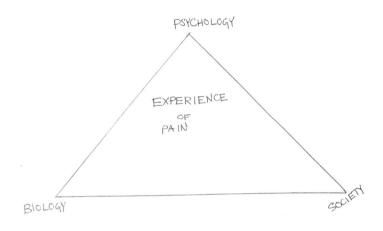

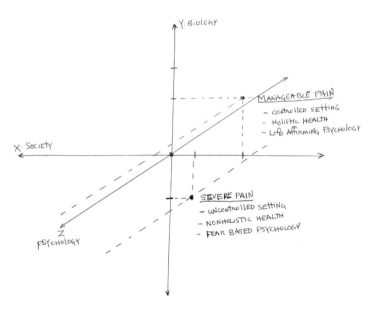

Chapter 6

MESSAGE TO THE BIRTH-WORKERS: WILL THE REVOLUTIONARY DOULAS PLEASE STAND UP

In the history of maternal wellness, it is beyond dispute that white men *and* women have played the most destructive role in furthering the systematic neglect, abuse, and killing of infants. From ancient Greece and Rome to medieval Europe and the "modern" west various forms of infanticide have exposed a psychotic streak among white women where the survival of their babies was sacrificed in the service of a violent, exploitative social order. In European Christian culture the act of overlaying or suffocating an infant in bed was so commonplace that it was considered a misdemeanor or as

Cheryl Meyer and Michelle Oberman state in their book *Mothers Who Kill Their Children*, "evidence of the prevalence of infanticide emerges from occasional references to the crime in medieval handbooks of penance ... This sin is included in a list of venial or minor sins, such as failing to be a good Samaritan or quarreling with one's wife." [16]After perfecting this total disregard for infants within their own territories white women carried the same procedures into the Black/ Afrikan world when they authorized the sale and trafficking of Black children around the continental United States. Contrary to popular myth, white women were instrumental to the growth of america's slave industry comprising at one time 40% of all slave owners.[17] This investment in the annihilation of Black families through slave auctions was often organized from the comfort of the white home through male agents and proxies, underscoring how despite the intensely patriarchal norms of white society, their women were granted equal access when it came to advancing the cultural genocide against Black people.

These two historical phenomena should be at the forefront of our minds as Black mothers and fathers when we recklessly allow white women to enter our birthing spaces as doulas, doulas-in-training, caregivers, or if we are assisting white women in giving birth to their children. How we give birth, like virtually everything else a

---

16 Meyer, Cheryl L., et al. *Mothers Who Kill Their Children Understanding the Acts of Moms from Susan Smith to the "Prom Mom"*. New York University Press, 2001.

17 Jones-Rogers, Stephanie E. *They Were Her Property: White Women as Slave Owners in the American South*. Yale University Press, 2020.

people do, comes out of a specific cultural background whose components must be jealously protected if those who practice its methods are serious about their genetic survival. **It is for this reason that Black doulas and mothers who grant access to white women in their practice—whether that be in the form of information sharing or being physically present during the birthing process—are engaged in an act of cultural negligence.** When Black men and women grant white women access to Black birthing spaces, spaces which should function as sanctuaries to insulate our communities from the spiritual toxins of mainstream white society, we are consenting to an invasion of the worst kind. Black mothers and children continue to die in western hospitals from preventable causes largely because of an irrational trust placed in white medical establishments and their technological/mechanized procedures of child labor.[18] The role of Black doulas should be to comprise that frontline of women who not only shield us from the technological aggression of white medicine but the cultural aggression embodied in white people's mere presence. This cultural aggression is manifest in the endless array of articles, books, apps, and instructional videos authored by white women which disregards the cultural particulars of Black birthing and postpartum practices. Nothing promotes the lie that white women are credible authorities on maternal wellness more effectively than the monopoly they exercise over the flow of all mainstream birthing information within and outside of their communities. As the genetic descendants of Afrikan women who were the world's pioneers in birth work it's

---

[18] According to recent studies, 2/3 of all Black maternal deaths in hospital settings are preventable.

imperative that we reclaim our collective power through policies designed to ensure our genetic survival. **At the core of this policy is a non-negotiable priority that says as long as Black women and children are dying at alarming rates at the hands of the white race, white women and their children should be of no concern to Black women.** Allegations that this is a racist position (which it proudly is) should not be a deterrent in following this path as all culturally literate, sovereign people make it a priority of the highest order to securitize those processes that are most essential to their long-term survival and what process is more essential to our survival than how we give birth and who we give birth in the presence of?

If you wouldn't allow a white woman to assist in the rearing of your child then you certainly shouldn't allow them to assist in the birthing of that child. We must be more intentional about creating life paths for our children that are free of the corruptive influences of our enemies. Seizing control of our children will never be complete as long as we allow those intent on their destruction to be in their presence. The plethora of media showing Black mothers being "assisted" by white birth workers highlights how much work needs to be done in racializing our critique of western birth practices. As Black fathers, we should be doing everything within our power to prevent the entry of these white birth workers into our homes. In the rare event that Black doulas are not available we should be making the necessary sacrifice and commitment to educate ourselves and assist the mothers of our children during labor. But achieving this degree of self-confidence and trust in self is only within reach once we sever the historical ties of codependence we have with our oppressors.

Chapter 7

PREVENTIVE MEASURES AGAINST POSTPARTUM DEPRESSION

Postpartum depression (PPD)—a mental illness that sets in after pregnancy characterized by mood swings, sadness, irritability, feelings of being overwhelmed, crying, and trouble sleeping[19]—is a widespread psychological issue that afflicts Black mothers across the United States with devastating consequences for the formation of balanced mother-child bonds. According to the National Alliance on Mental Illness, "PPD affects one in eight new mothers, but the risk is *significantly higher for new mothers of color*." The report goes on to add,

---

[19] Postpartum depression – Mayo Clinic

"while Black women are more likely to have PPD, they are less likely to receive help."[20] Causes for this disproportionate incidence of postpartum depression among Black mothers are diverse, ranging from economic hardship, stressful living environments, exposure to trauma, hunger, and lack of adequate healthcare accommodations. All of these social factors underscore how life within a white dominated culture poses severe psychological risk to the wellbeing of Black mothers. These risk factors must be militantly resisted by Black fathers to ensure the mothers of our children have the healthiest fourth trimester possible.

A more proactive, preventive approach in confronting this plague of the spirit would involve a look into how western birthing norms prepare the soil for postpartum depression to take root. Expanding upon the biological factors which contribute to PPD, Dr. Llaila Afrika notes how the cutting of the umbilical cord before the delivery of the placenta sets off a hormonal reaction which leads to postpartum depression:

"The cutting of the pulsating cord [the umbilical] causes the blood and the nutrients for the baby to stay in the placenta and become toxins. The mother's hormones trigger the destruction of the toxic placenta instead of her hormones triggering the ejection of the placenta out of the uterus. **Rejection of the placenta hormonally gets confused with rejection of the baby and this causes Postnatal Depression.**"

---

[20] Kilgoe, Ashley, "Addressing the Increased Risk of Postpartum Depression for Black Women"- National Alliance on Mental Illness (July 2021)

At the core of this hormonal rejection of the placenta is the shutting down of the release of oxytocin, the so-called "love hormone" released during and after labor responsible for the bonding between the mother and her baby. Oxytocin, along with other hormones, is found in high concentrations in the placenta.

OXYTOCIN: THE MASTER HORMONE TO FIGHT PPD

When it comes to building up biological defenses against the onset of postpartum depression oxytocin is the master hormone that Black mothers need to create healthy, enduring bonds with their babies. This hormone and neurotransmitter, which originates in the hypothalamus region of the brain, sends signals to the birthing mother (via the pituitary gland) that helps to regulate mood and behavior. Studies show that oxytocin levels in the mother reach their highest point during the labor process (3 pulses of oxytocin every 10 minutes toward the end of labor) and it plays an important role in controlling the length and pain of uterine contractions. Other major benefits to oxytocin for mothers during child labor include:

-Enhancement of mood and wellbeing
-Promotes friendly social relations
-Reduces anxiety and pain (a natural opiate)
-Reduces "fight or flight" response (fear)

-Increases relaxation and growth
-Increases sense of calmness and connection
-Helps mother forget labor pain

A large portion of the psychological distress associated with postpartum depression—feelings of alienation, that your child doesn't belong to you, disturbing fantasies that involve abandoning/harming the child, suicidal thoughts, etc.—are byproducts of a medical culture that has completely ignored the adaptive power of oxytocin in promoting mental wellness. For example, it is the hormonal release of oxytocin that warms the mother's chest for skin-to-skin contact after birth. This embrace between the mother and child seconds after birth is crucial in syncing the heartbeat and brain chemistry of the child with that of the mother (entrainment). Oxytocin also facilitates the delivery of the placenta, lowering risk of postpartum hemorrhage, making for a trauma free birth.

Too much of the dialogue around postpartum depression focuses exclusively on how to manage its effects rather than attacking its sources beforehand. Preemptively attacking the sources of PPD would most likely endanger the profits of Pitocin manufacturers (synthetic oxytocin) and the countless hospitals that provide a market for them to push their product. But as Black fathers we must grasp the truth that when we allow western medical practice to interfere with the natural chemistry of Black mothers we are opening the way for our homes to be infiltrated by not only the grief of postpartum depression but a number of other psychotic disorders which tear at the fabric of Black familyhood.

Therefore, as Black fathers the most effective preventive measure we can take in affording Black mothers the irreplaceable benefits of

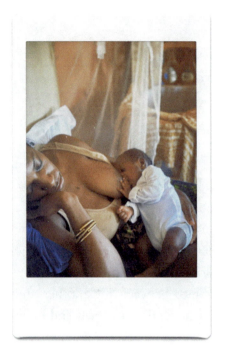
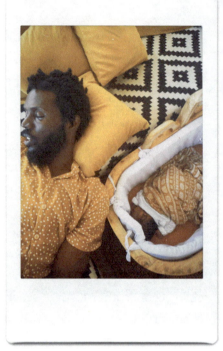
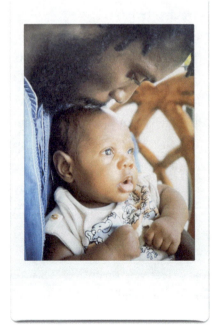
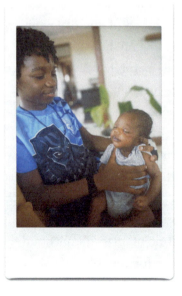

Jahi & his big brother Mikey

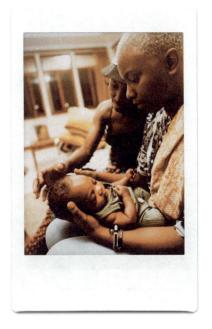

Our family visiting Jahi

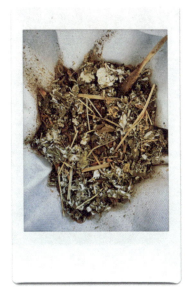

The placenta with seasoning

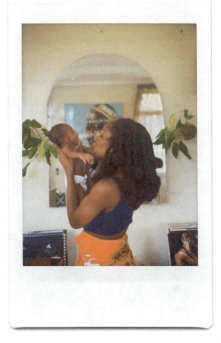

My wife singing to our son in the living room

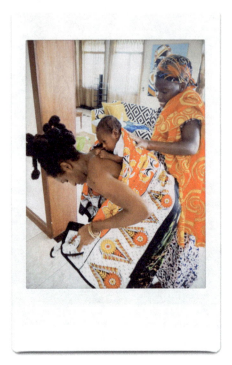

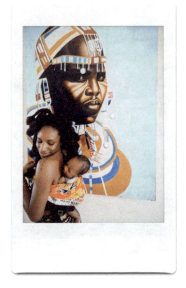

Shingazi teaching my wife how to tie Jahi to her
back with kitenge

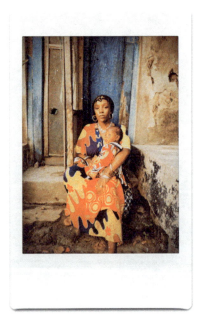

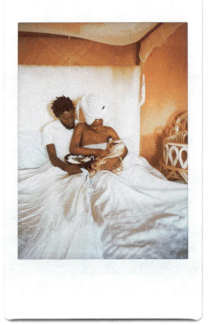

My wife and I with Jahi moments
after his birth

natural oxytocin is to strongly encourage them to keep as far away as possible from those spaces where its regenerating powers are devalued (hospitals). As a wide-ranging study on levels of oxytocin in the blood plasma of birthing mothers observes, "**Stressful and unfamiliar situations and surroundings may increase stress levels and decrease oxytocin release and PSNS [parasympathetic nervous system] activity.** Alternatively, situations perceived as safe, familiar, friendly and supportive by the mother are likely to do the opposite, and promote oxytocin release and PSNS activity."[21] [See Chapter on Protecting the Perimeter]

This dual approach—limiting medical interventions that compromise the natural integrity of the mother's hormonal response and actively working to stay away from places where natural birth is not protected—will contribute greatly in lowering the incidence of postpartum depression in Black mothers. The cumulative effect will be sovereign, mentally rehabilitated Black communities energized by a vision of their own making borne by a culture of their own design.

PITOCIN: THE ARTIFICIAL LOVE HORMONE

---

[21] Uvnäs-Moberg, K., Ekström-Bergström, A., Berg, M. *et al.* Maternal plasma levels of oxytocin during physiological childbirth – a systematic review with implications for uterine contractions and central actions of oxytocin. *BMC Pregnancy Childbirth* **19,** 285 (2019). https://doi.org/10.1186/s12884-019-2365-9

In an attempt to hi-jack the biochemical bond created by the love-hormone of oxytocin, modern day medical professionals have devised an artificial love hormone: Pitocin. First produced for medical practice in the 1950s based on the research of american biochemist Vincent du Vigneaud, the intravenous use of this hormone has become the method of choice in hospitals across the United States. According to The Journal of Perinatal Education nearly a third of mothers (31%) who gave birth vaginally used Pitocin to induce labor. This widespread acceptance of Pitocin use is occurring in an environment where its many negative effects on the physical and mental health of the mother and child are hidden. Peer-reviewed scientific studies have shown that Pitocin use, especially in high dosages, negatively impacts the mother in terms of her susceptibility to stress, regulation of mood, mothering behaviors, and lactation. Pitocin use also has been linked to long term psychological harm to the fetus. Negative effects of Pitocin use include:

-Longer and more painful contractions (justifying epidural use)
-Babies score lower score Apgar Test
-Higher chance of baby being submitted to NICU
-Reduction of lactation and feeding behavior in babies
-Twice as likely to cause attention deficit disorder in child
-Mother twice as likely to use formula after discharge after hospital

-Mother three times less likely to initiate breastfeeding within first 4 hours of labor[22]

For more information on the detrimental effects of Pitocin on the mother-child bond, an abundance of scientific research is available for reading. Some of the more informative titles are *Genomic and Epigenetic Evidence for Oxytocin Receptor Deficiency in Autism*, *Newborn Feeding Behavior Depressed by Intrapartum Oxytocin: A Pilot Study*, *Perinatal Pitocin as an Early ADHD Biomarker*, and *Fetal Exposure to Synthetic Oxytocin and the Relationship with Pre-feeding Cues Within One Hour of Post-Birth*.

COMPLEMENTARITY: OUR FIRST & LAST LINE OF DEFENSE

As important as the aforementioned biological factors are in preventing the onset of postpartum depression, nothing compares to the consistent, supportive presence of Black fathers in helping Black mothers navigate the emotional and psychological challenges of the postnatal period. It is now generally accepted that stressed relationships with the father of newborns carry negative psychological consequences for new mothers. What we should

---

[22] Bell, Aleeca F et al. "Beyond labor: the role of natural and synthetic oxytocin in the transition to motherhood." *Journal of midwifery & women's health* vol. 59,1 (2014): 35-42: quiz 108. doi:10.1111/jmwh.12101

understand as Black fathers is that when we devalue and fail to be the source of mental stability that our wives can rely upon in their hours of distress we are also indirectly depriving our baby of the mother he or she needs to develop a functional, balanced emotional self. In the Afrikan tradition fruitful bonds of complementarity between men and women served as a social safeguard against the possibility of the familial strain that comes about as a result of mental disorders such as postpartum depression. Afrikan-centered scholar Mwalimu Baruti provides a thorough definition of the sacred principle of complementarity as:

"A spiritual expression which, in practical Afrikan terms, means that we are speaking of intimate heterosexual relationships based on mutual trust, cultural and political alignment, belief in work (with divisions based on skills, abilities, and interests), repeated, honest, understanding forgiveness, having expressed heartfelt empathy and sympathy for each other, meaningfully communicating regularly, agreement on, and practice of sexual morality, family/child priority, fearless defense of each other and community, willing and receiving constructive criticism and last, but not least, mental, emotional, and physical fidelity."

Tapping into this spiritual core demands that we divorce ourselves from mainstream, europeanized conceptions of relationships that relegate the woman to an altogether inferior role. Balanced, complementarity relationships are both protective and reflective. By re-educating ourselves on the present dangers of a death-centered medical culture intent on robbing Black mothers of the divinity innate in childbirth we are erecting a protective shield against all outsiders and helping her to cultivate the needed environment for the promotion of life. On an anatomical level this is evident in the scientifically verified fact that breastfeeding triggers the release of oxytocin in the brain, aiding in the formation of a mother-child biochemical bond. This hormonal release substantially lowers the risk of postpartum depression.

In regard to the reflective power of complementarity, it compels the Black father to search deeply within the confines of his own psyche to reevaluate comfortable notions of commitment and intimacy. We truly discover our divine masculinity in those moments where we exercise the most patience and care with a vision toward long-term family growth. Along with consistent emotional support when it comes to encouraging our wives in their breastfeeding journey we also should be looking to figure out how we can alleviate the inevitable, physical strain that is a characteristic feature of the postnatal experience. Forms of physical and mental support that Black fathers engage in include:

-**Oiled foot and back massages**: Without words, we can communicate to our wives how appreciative we are of their physical sacrifice by aiding in their physical rejuvenation. As Maxim 21 of the Kemetic sage Ptahhotep eloquently states, "If you are excellent, you will establish your household and you shall love your wife with ardor. Fill her belly, clothe her back. **Ointment is the prescription for her limbs**. Gladden her heart as long as you live. She is a profitable field for her lord. You should not judge her, remove her from power, or restrain her. Her eye is her storm-wind when she sees. It means she shall endure in your house. When you repulse her, she is water. A vagina is what she gives for her condition.[23] What she questions is one who will make a canal for her."

-**Herbal foot baths**: Much like the foot and back massages, the herbal foot bath is meant to establish a mature intimacy that acknowledges the sacrifice of the mother of your children while also supplying her with the healing energy she needs to continue on her journey. It is ideal that herbs are handpicked from your front or backyard. Going through the process of customizing a foot bath for your wife will help strengthen your bond and build your confidence as not only a provider of material to your family but a source of mental and psychological renewal

- **Accommodating baby needs so that mother can get needed rest**: Caring for a newborn is an intrinsically time consuming responsibility that will inevitably involve late night feedings and disruption of normal sleeping cycles. This can lead to physical exhaustion and irritability in mothers. We can help undercut this by sacrificing more of our time to support the mother while she is breastfeeding, soothe the baby back to sleep when crying, changing the baby's diaper, etc. Anxiety can easily be created in mothers when they get the impression that the father is not equally invested in the

---

[23] Mario Beatty's translation as it appears in his essay *A new interpretation of the image of Women in Maxim 21 of the Instructions of Ptahhotep: A grammatical and cultural analysis.* Beatty interprets the line "a vagina is what she gives for her condition," as meaning, "The acceptance of the power (shm) of women is essential to the perpetuation of life."

childrearing process. Making this known by taking the initiative in this early period is a critical gesture of reassurance.

Postpartum depression, contrary to popular belief, does not make necessary the resort to antidepressants or other types of psychoactive drugs. Instead of addressing the underlying social and biological causes, these quick fixes merely manage the symptoms while nurturing dynamics of dependency that have the potential to wreak havoc on marital relations and the larger community within which healthy unions are formed. It is only when we aggressively resist the calculated assault on our families at the hands of hospitals, the pharmaceutical industry, and its supporters in the media that we can reclaim the mental wellness and child-centeredness that is the hallmark of Afrikan living.

Chapter 8

THE SPIRITUAL POWER OF PLACENTAL BIRTH

"Protection of the placenta is imperative because it may be used by evildoers to manipulate the life and energy of the newborn or its mother."[24]
—Tiffany D. Pogue

It's a scene familiar to many of us: a mother, after enduring hours of traumatic labor, stares exhaustedly at her baby held aloft by the physician. The pulsating umbilical cord is still intact. "Would you do the honors," asks the physician. In comes the father with blade in hand. He cuts the cord and blood spills out onto the sheets. This ritual has been misrepresented as a harmless initiation into

---

[24] Asante, Molefi Kete, and Ama Mazama. *Encyclopedia of African Religion*. SAGE, 2009.

fatherhood where in actuality it represents the destruction of the biological bond between the mother, father and child.

How did we get here? It begins with the demonization of the female anatomy, specifically the placenta, and its varied benefits in the creation of human bonds. This demonization was a sharp departure from what existed in many Afrikan and indigenous cultures where the spiritual power of the placenta was widely revered through the practice of placental (lotus) birth. In placental birth the placenta is recognized as a sacred symbol of the mother's blood while the umbilical cord symbolizes the conduit for the essence of the father to reach the child.

Instead of cutting the umbilical while the placenta is still inside of the uterus, the natural rhythms of the mother's body are allowed to expel the placenta. The placenta is then washed, placed in a bowl, and seasoned with herbs to be preserved for a number of days. The primary purpose of placental birth is to ensure that all the blood, oxygen, and vital nutrients from the organ enters the baby. This continuous supply of nutrients following birth (it is estimated that a third of the baby's blood is stored in the placenta) strengthens the immune system of the baby, lowering the probability of infectious disease. According to a 2018 case series report of placental birth the benefits of delayed cord clamping for babies born at term include, "increased hemoglobin levels at birth and improved iron stores for several months after birth, which may favorably affect infant development."

The report goes on to state, "for preterm infants, delayed clamping may improve transitional circulation and help increase red blood cell volume."[25]

Historical studies show that the care, preservation, and internment of the placenta was a common practice throughout the Afrikan, Asian, and indigenous world. Variations of placental reverence can be found in China, Japan, Malaysia, among the Mayans and Incas, the indigenous cultures of British Columbia and New Zealand, the Swahili people of East Afrika, and the melanin rich aboriginal populations of Australia. Meanwhile, in ancient Kemet, "the pharaoh led processions preceded by his actual placenta, fixed to the top of a long pole with a dangling umbilical cord." Other world cultures where placental birth is revered include the Igbo people of Nigeria, the Baganda, the Ngoni, the Edo, and Afrikan populations in the Caribbean from Jamaica to Haiti.

When this historical background is taken into consideration modern bias against placental birth as strange, "quackery", or a meaningless preservation of "waste" material is exposed for what it truly is: propaganda designed to convince Black mothers to relinquish the healing powers built up within their bodies. In the economic realm, this includes the confiscation and commodification of placental tissue for stem cell research. The average street value price for a placenta extracted from a new mother is $50,000. This is just

---

[25] Lotus Birth: A Case Series Report on Umbilical Nonseverance - Kimberly K. Monroe, Alexandra Rubin, Kerry P. Mychaliska, Maria Skoczylas, Heather L. Burrows, 2019

one of the several price tags "modern medical science" places on trauma. Some of the benefits of placental birth include:

-Increased blood flow to the baby

-The baby is not traumatized by the cutting of the cord

-Increases oxygen intake of the baby

-Increased nutrient flow to the baby

-Strengthening of the immune system of the baby

-Father is able to establish biochemical bond with child through massaging of placenta

-Ceremonial burial of placenta promotes spiritual wellness in home

-Promotes family bonding and sensitivity in how they relate to baby since cord is still attached for a number of days

-Makes respiratory transition of baby from breathing in the amniotic fluids of the womb to breathing in air easier.

OUR PLACENTAL BIRTH STORY

When my wife and I decided to birth our son via placental birth we knew that this was a sharp break from mainstream birthing culture (and even natural birthing culture in some respects) but we also understood that reneging on this commitment would mean depriving our son of essential nutrients that were impossible to replace. Following the birth of our son and the delivery of the placenta (naturally without the use of Pitocin) it was gently washed in water and placed into a wooden bowl lined with cotton to absorb excess fluid. We then seasoned the placenta with a mix of herbs—yoni steam herbs and red raspberry leaf—to mask the smell. The placenta was flipped, re-washed, and re-seasoned once per day.

As the placenta was washed I massaged the thin tissue to eliminate any blood clots and facilitate more flow through the umbilical. This massaging process is critical and ideally should be carried out by the father because through the father's touch he is establishing a bond with the baby. Remember the placenta is just as much a part of the newborn as his kidney, liver, or bladder.[26] Therefore, it's imperative

---

[26] Osteopath Dr. Luca Daini documents in the 2011 book *Lotus Birth* the placental birth of his daughter and how the CRI (Cranial Rhythmic Impulse) of the placenta attached to her navel matched the CRI of his daughter. This led him to conclude, "it was as if the infant's body and the placenta were one unit, partaking in the same 'breathing exercise.'"

we treat it with the appropriate tenderness and respect to nurture a strong connection.

In placental birth the umbilical cord naturally separates from the navel. When that point nears, it will be obvious. The pulsating white cord will become dry, brown, and shriveled. In four days, our son's umbilical cord pumped all the vital nutrients needed into his body and neatly detached. The break off point at his navel was so precise that when we took him to the local clinic to be weighed one member of the medical staff asked my wife, in clear disbelief, "is your husband a doctor?"

The successful completion of our placental birth was pivotal in instilling in us a confidence that we were intellectually equipped and possessed the right amount of discipline to safeguard the immune health of our son. In the last ceremony of this practice it is customary to bury the organ. We chose to bury our placenta in a potted plant on the balcony just outside our bedroom. As we raked handfuls of dirt over the decayed organ my wife said, "thank you for keeping our baby alive." It took me a few seconds to realize that she was talking to the placenta, the living spirit that came out of her. Through this meticulously designed, Afrikan-centered ritual both my wife and I received an education in how to be responsible stewards of life. Our son was able to part ways with his primary source of sustenance without the trauma of having his oxygen supply depleted or the long-term effects of a nutritional deficiency.[27] We, as a family,

---

[27] Elizabeth Noble, cited in Anand Khushi's essay titled, "The Placenta and Cord in Other Cultures," observes, "In primitive tribes the placenta was often called the 'double', 'soul', 'secret helper', or 'brother', and was buried or placed in a tree or on top of a pole." – *Lotus Birth* (2011)

were able to experience the beauty of loss without grief and death as nothing more than a transition. For me this is what it means to embrace the responsibility of Black fatherhood and unlike the premature cutting of cords this was a genuine honor.

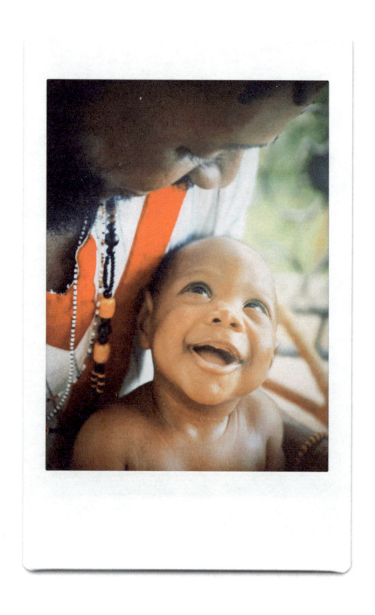

Chapter 9

FATHER BONDING TECHNIQUES

"As for the *Kra*, Field defines it as 'the spirit which makes the difference between a dead body and a living body.' Meaning, the *kra* is an 'invisible double' and the essence of life, which cannot leave the body 'without causing sickness and death.' The *kra* originates with the father, while the body and blood have their source with the mother."

-Anthony Ephirim Donkor

In the Akan spiritual system of West Afrika newborns are understood to be a combination of the blood of the mother and the spirit of the father. The blood of the newborn, *Mogya*, is derived from the eggs of the mother whereas the spirit of the newborn, *Sunsum*, is inherited through the father's semen. While the *Mogya* (blood) of the mother represents, "the physical component of the personality", the *Sunsum* (semen) represents the "unique masculine agency," of the father— "the unifying and protective component of every family unit." This holistic conception of the newborn as a bio-spiritual expression of the natural powers of its parents should motivate us to reconsider the central role of father-child bonding in laying the groundwork for healthy family dynamics. For the purposes of this book, the role of the father is paramount.

The first fact that fathers must understand when it comes to bonding with their children is that the bonding process begins prenatally long before the child is born. Studies have shown that babies begin responding to voices in the womb at 25 weeks. Talking to your baby before its arrival date will not only give him or her an early introduction to your personality but it will also prepare us mentally to embrace the responsibilities of bonding months in advance. Maintaining a calm, functional relationship with the mother of our children during pregnancy is also critical in bonding with our children. When intimate relationships are overwhelmed by stress, a chemical release is triggered in the brain that can negatively affect the overall biochemistry of the mother. These stress hormones are then transmitted via the mother's amniotic fluid to the baby increasing the likelihood of early health complications in the newborn. Incidences of asthma, preterm birth, infant mortality, ADHD, cardiovascular disease, and low birthweight have all been linked to undue stress imposed on the mother during the prenatal period.[28] We must understand that the biological bond between the mother and the

---

[28] "Too Much Stress for the Mother Affects the Baby through Amniotic Fluid." *UZH*, Universität Zürich, 13 Dec. 2017, https://www.media.uzh.ch/en/Press-Releases/2017/stress-hormones-in-amniotic-fluid.html.

child throughout the entirety of the perinatal period (three trimesters of pregnancy and one year postpartum) is so close that any psychological, emotional, or physical stress imposed on the mother is simultaneously imposed on the infant.

As Black fathers, we are indirectly bonding with our children in how we attend to the emotional, physical, and psychological needs of their mother. The early infancy of your child's life is a time when the biological complexity of the mother is key in organizing their many physical and psychological traits from their cognitive-emotional development and immune health to the rhythmic frequency of their heart and breath. In many subtle and not so subtle ways the mother is telling a story to our children, through the chemistry of her body, about us, their fathers. We must do all within our power to ensure that the story her body tells is one from which our children can draw positive inspiration. This is the decoded meaning of the Afrikan proverb, "It takes a breast for a child to know its mother and it takes a mother for a child to know its father." Dysfunctional, bond-damaged relationships with the mother of our children inevitably breeds dysfunctional, bond-damaged relationships with our children themselves. There is no way around this truth.

Apart from this indirect method of father-child bonding, more direct approaches are available as well. Among these perhaps the most important is the establishment of early skin-to-skin contact with the baby. In valuing skin-to-skin contact we are nurturing an emotional bond with our child that could not be accomplished by non-physical means. A 2017 Taiwanese Ministry of Health study evaluating the benefits of skin-to-skin contact among Taiwanese fathers, "[confirmed] the positive effects of SSC [skin-to-skin contact] interventions on the infant behavior of fathers in terms of exploring, talking, touching, and caring and on the father-neonate attachment relationship at three days postpartum." The clinical implications drawn from this research included an acknowledgment that, "expanding the skin-to-skin care approach to fathers may be an effective healthcare strategy that **helps new fathers develop self-confidence and adopt a more positive outlook on their transition into fatherhood.**"[29] Here we have scientific proof that skin-to-skin contact has mutual benefits for the father and the child. In other words, the more we invest, through our actions, in bonding with our children the deeper the transformation on the psychological level. As with all holistic teachings, skin-to-skin contact is about bringing the body and mind into proper alignment.

SEX DURING PREGNANCY: A PSCYHOSPIRITUAL RISK FACTOR

One of the easiest and most effective ways to culturally decimate a population of people is to colonize their sexual appetites. Once those in power have seized control of our lower regions every decision we make, from our diets, to how we conduct our relationships, to the amount of time we invest in rearing our children are compromised. In the West, this reality is evident in the mainstream advocacy of sexual intercourse as an acceptable, and even "healthy", practice for

---

[29] Chen, Er-Mei, et al. "Effects of Father-Neonate Skin-to-Skin Contact on Attachment: A Randomized Controlled Trial." *Nursing Research and Practice*, Hindawi Publishing Corporation, 2017, https://www.ncbi.nlm.nih.gov/pmc/articles/PMC5282438/.

pregnant women. This norm can only persist in a society that has completely de-spiritualized all aspects of maternal health to the point where the actions of the parents are discounted in the formation of the personality of the baby. According to a study conducted in Lisbon, Portugal evaluating the sexual activity of 188 women between the ages of 17 and 40, "80% of women reported some kind of sexual activity during their third trimester. And, 39% reported sexual intercourse during their birth week." While statistics are not available on the prevalence of perinatal sex in the United States it is generally accepted as, "perfectly safe" and "normal", a byproduct of a medical culture narrowly focused on physiological outcomes at the expense of holistic wellness. Even today those at the frontlines of maternal health, Black doulas and birth workers, have been misled into believing that sex during pregnancy is normal and has no adverse effects on the baby. We must understand that this perspective is borne from a white-dominated culture that devalues life and has infiltrated even our most respected realms of knowledge in the Black community.

As descendants of Afrika in an anti-Afrikan society it is imperative that we develop a healthy distrust for anything white society deems "safe" or "normal" as what is beneficial for their culture is always destructive to ours. Dr. Llaila Afrika reminds us of both the spiritual and psychological dangers of sex during pregnancy in his magnum opus *Afrikan Holistic Health*. Describing a Black population manipulated into becoming "sexual clowns," he identifies sex during pregnancy as a peculiar behavior exclusive to whites throughout most of world history:

"In traditional cultures (non-Caucasian), during the breastfeeding period of time sex was not allowed. **In fact, no animal ... [has] sex while pregnant except [in] traditional Caucasian culture.** Sex while the female is pregnant changes the hormone and nutrient of the fetus, alters the biochemistry of the female and causes sympathetic stress. This rule of sexual abstinence protects the species and creates a sexual system that sustains a culture."[30]

Sex during pregnancy is also destructive to the ratio of hormones in the mother. Specifically, when mothers engage in sex during pregnancy the levels of progesterone in her body decreases while the levels of testosterone increase. This increase in testosterone in the mother then contributes to an excess of aggression in the baby while it is still in the womb. Basic reasoning tells us that nothing is more corrosive to the cultivation of healthy bonds than the multiple forms of aggression we encounter within our homes whether it be domestic violence, verbal abuse, sexual abuse, or neglect.

From a cultural-historical perspective our Afrikan forebears understood the supreme importance of practicing abstinence during pregnancy. Renowned scholar of Afrikan culture Ama Mazama observes in the *Encyclopedia of African Religion*, "among the Gurunsi of southern Burkina Faso and northern Ghana, sexual relations are prohibited between a pregnant woman and her husband beginning around the third month of the pregnancy. "[31] It should be recognized that this practice, which represents one aspect of a broader ritual

---

[30] *African Holistic Health* [Revised and Expanded 7th Edition] (2011) – Dr. Llaila O. Afrika

[31] Asante, Molefi Kete, and Ama Mazama. *Encyclopedia of African Religion*. SAGE, 2009.

system called the *legume* ritual, is a more liberal counterpart to other norms on the continent that forbids any sexual intercourse between a mother and the father of their child at the point of the pregnancy's discovery regardless of term. How far have we strayed from basic principles of Afrikan living when we not only advocate sexual intercourse during pregnancy but *celebrate* it as a method of inducing labor?!

Disowning the hedonistic, pleasure driven ideologies of white society and returning to holistic, Afrikan-centered concepts of sexuality[32] which factors in the psychological, spiritual, and cultural dimensions of sex requires we exercise a level of sexual discipline where we think with our brains instead of our genitals. In doing this we will be making a desperately needed contribution in the protection of the emotional core of our children. Out of this emotional core comes the ingredients necessary for building meaningful, spiritual bonds with them. Only then can we be the "unifying and protective component," of our families that our ancestors ordained us to be.

Proactive measures that can be taken to occupy ourselves during this critical period include:

---

[32] In his book on the Akan spiritual system, *African Spirituality: On Becoming Ancestors* Anthony Ephirim-Donkor describes Afrikan male sexuality as follows: "There is an aspect of a male—likeness—that is imbued with a woman resulting in pregnancy. Therefore, there is more than a physical aspect to *sunsum*: it is transferal, meaning a man takes more than his physical nature, strength, or characteristic attributes into a sexual encounter—he takes his essence (su), presence and glory into a copulative encounter." (p. 54)

-Practice sex sublimation or the channeling of sexual energies towards creative endeavors in the form of art, production, intellectual work, etc. to elevate yourself to a higher level of consciousness (See Muata Ashby's *Sacred Sexuality* for more information on this).

-Intense research on prenatal and postpartum health so that you can enter fatherhood as informed as possible (this book is a great start).

-Finding creative ways to foster intimacy with your partner outside of sex (See Chapter on Postpartum Depression)

-Investing in substantive, meaningful conversation with partner about their mental outlook, pregnancy challenges, and vision for the future

-Plan a getaway together

-Start a small project together that you both are passionate about

-Cook healthy, nutritious meals together

-Plan a thoughtful surprise/experience that she would value

-Be present and involved in all maternity related activities

-Understand that sacrificing at least a year of sexual abstinence is a small sacrifice for helping to lay the basis for lifelong mental and emotional stability for your child.

Ultimately, sex during pregnancy evidences, more than any other behavior prior to birth, a fundamental selfishness in regard to the welfare of the child. When a baby is in utero it exists within a delicate ecosystem of life full of amniotic fluids, nutrients, and spiritual forces that are conducive to its full growth and development. When the parents choose to have sexual intercourse during pregnancy they are violating the equilibrium of life that exists within the mother's womb by introducing useless sperm cells that do not lead to the production of more life. In essence, the man who ejaculates in the womb of a pregnant woman is polluting her creative/spiritual core with lifeless, lustful energy. Afrikan architectural symbolism has always equated the life-giving capacities of the mother's womb with the generative logic that operates within the Afrikan home. This is the reason why Afrikan homes are traditionally designed in the form of a circle. The circular shape is meant to symbolize the gestational center of the norms, values, culture, and spiritual system of those who occupy the home. Therefore, failing to protect the womb by refraining from sexual intercourse during pregnancy is tantamount to failure to protect the home. As long as we remain captive to these pleasure-driven ideologies that place the self-gratification of the parents over and above the holistic wellness of the child our homes and our communities will be faced with the ruinous effects of dysfunctional families and general powerlessness.

Chapter 10

CRYING: OUR BABY'S ONLY DIALOGUE

Fathers navigating the challenges of early infant care must understand the value of patience in attending to the needs of their baby. Since infants have yet to develop the gift of speech crying is the sole means through which they communicate both their physiological and psychological desires. In this regard, your baby's cries should not be a cause for panic or stress. Rather these cries should be seen as an attempt to engage in dialogue with the parent. Out of this dialogue emerges a deep, biochemical connection. Crying, when disconnected from trauma or clear injury, is not only natural but a positive thing when parents are patient and adequately informed in how to respond. According to a study in the *Journal of Child Psychology and Psychiatry* when a baby cries, it stimulates a greater sensitivity in the mother—what is called "maternal sensitivity"—aiding in the "social-emotional development," of the infant. More interestingly, the study noted that, "compared to formula-feeding mothers, breastfeeding mothers have increased parasympathetic nervous system modulation, greater vascular stress response, lower perceived stress levels, and fewer depressive symptoms."[33] These neurological processes are all triggered and mediated by the cries of the baby or as a Press Association article on breastfeeding published in the UK *Guardian* states, "crying and irritability were likely to act as an 'honest signal' of nutritional need during pregnancy, when a lot of energy was needed for growth."[34] Taking this in mind, the frequent crying among infants is less of an indication of something being wrong with them than something being wrong with the parents, namely a lack of patience and understanding of natural processes.

Rallying against this scientific data, formula companies market their products as beneficial to new mothers because formula-fed babies on average sleep longer. When the infant sleeps longer, formula companies argue, the mother has more time to rest. For example, Australian based formula company Novolac Sweet Dreams — "sweet dreams" being an overt reference to the promise of

---

[33] Kim, Pilyoung, et al. "Breastfeeding, Brain Activation to Own Infant Cry, and Maternal Sensitivity." *Journal of Child Psychology and Psychiatry, and Allied Disciplines,* U.S. National Library of Medicine, Aug. 2011, https://www.ncbi.nlm.nih.gov/pmc/articles/PMC3134570/.

[34] "Breastfed babies show more challenging temperaments, study finds." *Guardian*, Press Association (2012)

extended sleep—baits consumers by saying that their product will guarantee that babies get extra sleep. Absent from this deceptive marketing scheme is that prolonged sleeping patterns in newborns is a physiological response to constipation. Studies also show extended, deep sleep is linked to a higher probability of SIDs (sudden infant death syndrome). As a result, parents sacrifice the health of their children and critical bonding time for the sake of a few extra hours of sleep. Like many other western perspectives on neonatal care, this attempt to needlessly extend the sleeping hours of babies selfishly prioritizes the comfort of the parent above the health of the child or the heart-brain connection needed to facilitate true wellness. As Black fathers, we should be willing to lose some hours of sleep to ease their cries and, by connection, bond with our children. Soothing our babies can take many forms from protecting the environment to facilitate breastfeeding and establishing skin-to-skin contact to singing them songs. Whatever method of care we apply, it's important we never look at crying, in itself, as the issue but rather how we respond to it. Crying is, at its core, a survival mechanism that ensures our baby gets the nutrients and care it needs. This is why all infants in the mammalian world communicate with their mothers through their cries. It is only among humans that we look upon this natural process as "problematic." Yet, as fathers we are biologically wired to respond to this desire for closeness. Evidence of this wiring is apparent in our brain chemistry; hence, "researchers found that within 49 thousandths of a second of a recorded cry being played, the periaqueductal gray — an area deep in the midbrain that has long been linked to urgent, do-or-die behaviors — had blazed to attention."[35] In this context, the widespread usage of pacifiers (artificial nipples) should be reinterpreted as an attempt to shut down the dialogue between the parent and the child by inhibiting the chemical release in the brain of the parent. Other negative side effects of pacifier use include[36]:

-Misalignment of baby's teeth
-Increased likelihood of middle ear infections
-Disruption of breastfeeding
-Creation of unhealthy dependence on pacifiers
-Increase likelihood of gastrointestinal and respiratory problems

Ultimately, the usage of pacifiers, baby formula, and the growing chorus of complaints against crying babies is evidence of a mainstream media culture intent on demonizing infants as nuisances whose only redeemable attribute is their cuteness. The cliché scene of the inconsolable baby crying on a plane, bus, or in a crowded movie theater is the mental image of choice underlying this attitude. Disconnecting from this culture of consumerist individualism that places a low value on patience and parent-child bonding is crucial for us to rise to the occasion to be the source of true comfort in which our children can confide.

---

[35] Angier, Natalie. "A Baby Wails, and the Adult World Comes Running." *The New York Times*, The New York Times, 4 Sept. 2017, https://www.nytimes.com/2017/09/04/science/crying-babies-animals.html.

[36] Sexton, Sumi M., and Ruby Natale. "Risks and Benefits of Pacifiers." *American Family Physician*, 15 Apr. 2009, https://www.aafp.org/afp/2009/0415/p681.html.

When pacifiers aren't at hand mothers are stereotypically portrayed as disheveled, exhausted, and stressed beyond normal limits by the wailing of their children. This portrayal, like all else in western societies, evidences a fundamental disregard for the emotional and spiritual complexity of infant communication habits and how a thorough analysis of these habits could benefit parents in their childrearing methods.

When an infant begins to cry, it is important that parents not respond to it in a panicked state. The postpartum period, while separate from the pregnancy period, is no less delicate an environment for your newborn. The varied emotional, biological, and spiritual energies that the infant absorbed in utero continues to flow in the postpartum period. In many ways, the family home can be symbolically interpreted as an external womb where the early spiritual development of the newborn takes place. In this external womb of the home the infant is constantly internalizing and translating the energies or aura of the people in its immediate environment. This heightened sensitivity is central to how the infant expresses itself and how it responds to others. Whether we know it or not, our babies are reading us and as parents we should know how to read them.

This being the case, it is critical that parents are able to make the distinction between the communication signal of their baby (crying) and the entity that this signaling system is directing you to (the baby itself). When we respond to our baby's cries calmly and intentionally we are offering non-verbal assurance to him or her that they are safe. In other words, we are most equipped to quell the cries of our baby when quelling their cries is no longer the primary objective but actually *seeing* your child and understanding its needs.

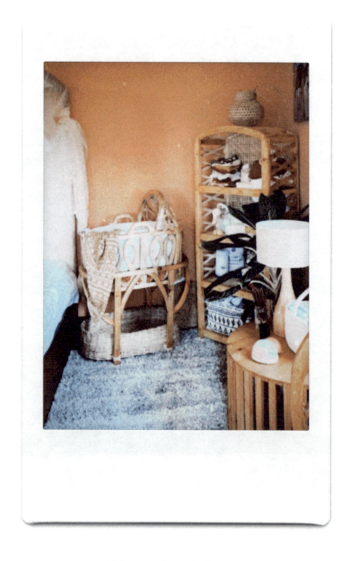

Jahi's corner in our bedroom

Chapter 11

INTENTIONAL UNMEDIATED TOUCHING

When dealing with newborns it is imperative that we as parents understand the central role of closeness and touch in our baby's spiritual and emotional education. When touch and closeness is given its proper role, the parent is replicating the environmental benefits of the mother's womb in the home. Failing to do this runs the risk of severely impairing the overall development of our children, creating a breeding ground for behavioral issues later in their lives. For this reason, a frame of reasoning and a method of interacting with our children in ways that are conducive to their long-term growth is in order. The best method for stimulating spiritual growth within our children is through *intentional unmediated touching*.

Intentional unmediated touching bridges the psychological/ emotional demands of childrearing with the biological/physical demands by centering the ability of the parent to positively focus their life-giving energies on the child as the decisive factor in healthy childrearing. To touch your baby intentionally means to engage with them in such a way that it aligns with the mother or father's understanding of the baby's many needs and, significantly, that parent's determined role within the family. A mother who is practicing intentional touching of her baby will breastfeed her child without hesitation because she is acutely aware of not only her responsibility to the infant as an abundant source of emotional nourishment and nutrition but her broader responsibility to the Afrikan community as the engine for the reproduction of Afrikan culture. Likewise, a father who is engaged in intentional touching will never de-link his physical interactions with his baby from his broader social role as a protector and spiritual guardian of his child.

This intentional approach to touching can only be of maximum benefit to the Afrikan family when it is unmediated by any device, gadget, or consumer item. We touch our babies in ways that transcend physical limits when we eliminate all barriers to the energy transfer (emotion) between the parent and the child introduced by the dominant white culture. Car seats, harnesses, strollers, high chairs, and other unnecessary accessories that are marketed to parents of newborns are all mediating devices designed to bastardize and corrupt this unmediated parent-child bond.

It is in the cultural DNA (asili) of the white populations of the world to look upon all relationships, familial included, as conflictual. It is for this reason that their culture demands the invention of these mediating devices—to *mediate* the conflict between the parent and the child. As Afrikan people who are inheritors of a tradition such as a the Kindezi system of the Bantu people which formalized the art of touching as an essential ingredient in healthy, holistic child rearing, we should look upon these so called advances in white technology as dangerous to Afrikan living. All objects purchased for or used in conjunction with our babies should be adopted for the explicit purpose that they meaningfully advance the welfare of our child, not facilitate the "me-time" for the adult. In other words, unless the technology being used contributes in those areas most crucial for the baby's physical/emotional health—touch and closeness—then that technology should be disposed of.

By comparison we can look at the white technology of the stroller and compare it to the Afrikan technology of the kitenge. While the stroller eliminates all touch and closeness between the parent and the child, the kitenge (by allowing the mother to tie the infant to her back) advances the closeness between the parent and the child while also advancing the touch to the point that the baby can listen to its mother's heartbeat. In the technically simple but spiritually complex usage of the kitenge we have a textbook example of intentional, unmediated touching. Embedded in this interaction is a transfer of emotion that could not have possibly taken place with the use of a stroller. Perhaps this is the most troubling fact when it comes to the attachment among Afrikans in the western world to the manufactured items of white industry. The end result of this negative socialization is the parent accepts consumerist mediated contact as the only viable means to communicate with their child. Under this logic mere "contact" replaces the more emotionally potent implications of touch and systematic neglect becomes habitual. One dramatic example of consumerist mediated contact is in the widespread use of pacifiers. Through the pacifier, the parent is withholding the attention that babies need and in effect denying the very existence of the child. More than instilling in the infant feelings of happiness, attention (when compassionately directed) affirms the existence of our infant children. In the west, where all attention directed toward our babies competes with the selfish desires of adults, there is bound to be a great deal of deprivation or attention-deficits. Tragically, the end result is a society defined along the lines of parent-centeredness and not child-centeredness. For Afrikans this is equivalent to cultural suicide.

Personally, when our son arrived we were adamant that the richly rewarding features of holistic bonding would not be sacrificed upon the altar of consumerism. Everything we need to sustain our son physically and emotionally fits into a small corner in our bedroom. Apart from the financial benefits of not having to expend valuable resources on items that would do nothing to promote our son's growth, this conscientious decision expanded the amount of space for us to create zones of intentional unmediated touching. We understood that nothing could replace the positive contribution of letting our son know that his parents are always available to acknowledge him as an integral member of the home and not a burden to be passed off onto the gadgets of our enemies. When we come into this deeper understanding of our role and responsibilities as parents we open doors to new ways of living and being that are nurturing to all.

Chapter 12

PARENT CENTEREDNESS VS. CHILD CENTEREDNESS

Within traditional Afrikan societies child-centeredness or the organizing of society around the physical and spiritual needs of the child was and remains essential to long term collective development. When the multiple needs of the child are attended to the groundwork for a functional civilization is established along with the creation of selfless individuals who are willing to make sacrifices on behalf of the whole. Since the rise of western industrial societies this child-centered approach to social organization has been brutally marginalized. In its place has arisen a highly individualistic and pleasure based ideology of parent-centeredness. Under the rule of parent-centered institutions the "me-time" of the mother shares space with time otherwise devoted to the nourishment of the child. At its core parent-centeredness is about producing bond-damaged children by detaching the emotional and psychological wellness of the mother from that of the child. All of the spiritually beneficial processes that come about through the mother's ability to replicate the womb state for her child are abandoned in the service of narrowly personal and nonproductive interests (shopping, night clubbing, extravagant vacations, brunch dates, etc.)

For mothers who aspire to escape the corruptive influence of a parent-centered culture it is critical they begin valuing the irreplaceable role of breastmilk, touch, and closeness in setting the biological and environmental standard for neonatal wellness. Breastmilk, particularly through the nipple, transfers the emotions, temperature, and temperament of the mother while touch and closeness is the environmental context in which this spiritual/cultural transmission takes place. By prioritizing milk, touch, and closeness mothers and fathers are bringing a holistic perspective to their childrearing methods that looks upon the conscious management of comforting environments, and not just nutritional supply, as integral to the early development of infants. University of Wisconsin psychologist Harry Harlow explored this question of comfort in a series of lab experiments on rhesus monkeys in the 1950s. In these experiments, Harlow placed "orphaned" (kidnapped) monkeys in isolation chambers to evaluate their behavioral development in conditions of maternal bonding and maternal deprivation. Each chamber was equipped with two surrogate mothers, one of which was made out of wire with a feeding bottle attached and the other was covered in cloth without a bottle attached. Interestingly, the experiment demonstrated that when the monkey was made to choose between the milk-supplying wire mother and the non-milk supplying cloth mother the monkey spent the overwhelming amount of its time attached to the cloth mother. The explanation for this behavior was that despite the fact that the wire mother supplied the infant monkey with milk in the psychology of an infant comfort—milk, touch, and closeness—is the leading motive and desire in behavior. In fact, comfort was so crucial that some of the monkeys in the experiment reportedly died from the loneliness of maternal deprivation. Other adverse effects of withholding comfort from the infant monkeys included acts of self-mutilation, non-nutritional sucking (pacifiers), an inability to form stable heterosexual relationships, a reduced sense of independence and security, and a lack of confidence. On the matter of developing confidence those monkeys that were not deprived of the comforting touch of the cloth mother bravely defended their space from external threats while those who were deprived, when faced with a threat, could only cower in fear.

From this observation, we arrive at a basic principle about the importance of comforting mother-child bonds, namely that in societies that work to suppress the formation of healthy, whole bonds the general character of its people is one of dependency, cowardice, and insecurity. Conversely, in those societies which elevate mother-child bonding through the promotion of breastfeeding, co-sleeping, baby wearing, and other unmediated forms of contact the defining character traits of those people will be confidence, self-sufficiency, and courage. Yet building the sovereign, self-reliant communities needed to truly nurture our children will not be possible unless we rise above the social engineering of our enemies and the destructive technologies they use to accomplish their goals.

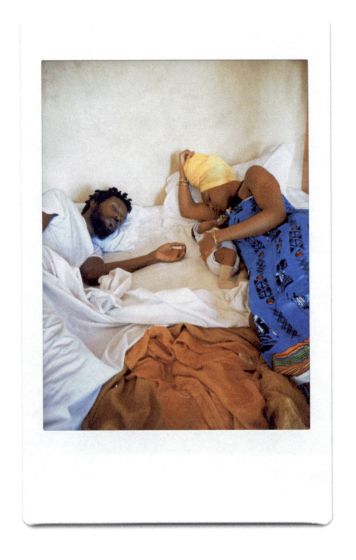

My wife, Jahi, and I co-sleeping

Chapter 13

THE BEAUTIFUL BENEFITS
OF CO-SLEEPING

There is a popular Afrikan proverb that states, "what the parents discuss in the evening the child will talk about in the morning." This simple adage is meant to highlight how the psychological and emotional state of the parents leave an indelible mark on the mind of their offspring. Harmonious, functional relationships between mothers and fathers is therefore indispensable within the Afrikan context. On a more literal level, this proverb can be taken as an ancestral recognition of how closeness between parents and their children is one of the defining features of the Afrikan family concept. Co-sleeping—the time-honored practice of parents sharing a bed with their infant child—is a relevant example of this closeness in the realm of early child care.

Despite mountains of propaganda instilling fear in new parents with the image of a sleeping mother or father rolling over on their baby and suffocating it to death, scientific analysis of this topic has yielded information favorable to co-sleeping as essential to the early development of infants. "When parents and babies sleep together, their heart rates, brain waves, sleep states, oxygen levels, temperature and breathing influence one another."[37] This was just one of many findings included in a study carried out by University of Notre Dame anthropologist James McKenna, who also concluded that co-sleeping initiated a neurological process called "synaptogenesis" or "the rapid growth of connections between neurons in newborns." Beneficial aspects of co-sleeping are also equitably shared between the mother and the father.

According to research conducted in the Philippines comparing fathers who co-slept with their babies to those who did not ("solitary sleepers"), co-sleeping fathers were found to have experienced measurable decreases in daytime (diurnal) testosterone levels.[38] This dip in testosterone translated into more sensitivity and greater paternal investment on the part of the father. These results were arrived at on the basis of the scientifically verifiable fact that high

[37] Divecha, Diana. "How Cosleeping Can Help You and Your Baby." *Greater Good*, https://greatergood.berkeley.edu/article/item/how_cosleeping_can_help_you_and_your_baby

[38] Gettler, Lee T, et al. "Does Cosleeping Contribute to Lower Testosterone Levels in Fathers? Evidence from the Philippines." *PloS One*, Public Library of Science, 2012, http://www.ncbi.nlm.gov/pmc/articles/PMC3434197/.

testosterone levels, "may interfere with paternal investment." Other major findings in this study, "the first to test for relationships between co-sleeping and paternal physiology", include:

-Fathers who co-sleep with their babies contribute to greater self-esteem, greater socialization skills, higher academic performance and lower incidence of delinquency in their children.

-Co-sleeping fathers had an, "evolved capacity to respond to childcare and direct contact with children."

Moreover, fathers, mothers, and infants will get more overall sleep if they co-sleep rather than if they have the infant sleep separately.

On the Afrikan continent one of the more widespread forms of co-sleeping is in the practice of baby-wearing or wrapping of the baby in *kitenge* (East Afrikan fabric) and securely tying them to the mother's back. In addition to positioning the baby so that it can be lulled to sleep by the heartbeat of the mother this practice also replicates the spatial experience of the mother's womb. The motion of the mother combined with the cocoon-like state of the infant is ideal for promoting closeness and calm in the baby. This is why mothers who practice baby wearing have little to any difficulty getting their baby to fall asleep. It's important not to confuse this traditional practice with the use of harnesses which attaches the baby to the front the parent with the baby's arms and legs freely exposed (traditional baby wearing hides the face of the baby in the early months. This allows the baby to experience the dark ambience of the mother's womb). Remember, the mother's touch is the decisive factor in baby wearing so you want to ensure the baby is at least in a position to hear the pulse of the parent. While baby wearing can be practiced by mothers and fathers it is imperative that it be primarily done with mothers as this biochemical bond should take precedent over the father-child bond during infancy.

Why then, with such an abundance of empirical data attesting to the benefits of co-sleeping for mothers and fathers, does this practice remain a "controversial" issue in the west? The answer to this lies in the history of western societies and its associated culture characterized by a fixation on death and psychosexual disorder. The familiar fear of co-sleeping being a prelude to infant death by asphyxiation originated in the caves and hills of northern europe (Paris, Brussels, Munich, and London) where, "Catholic priests heard confessions from destitute women who had 'overlain' onto their newborns, suffocating them in a desperate attempt to limit their family size ..." So socially prevalent were these exercises in european infanticide that, "the church ordered that babies should sleep in a separate cradle until the age of three."[39] This religious prohibition against co-sleeping received a boost from the european psychological establishment when Sigmund Freud recommended against parent-child co-sleeping since, "babies would be harmed if they were exposed to the parent's sexuality." On the behavioral science end of the psychological spectrum Dr. John Watson advocated babies sleep in separate rooms from parents in order not to ruin them with too much affection, or as he put it, "never hug and kiss them ... shake hands with them in the morning." It is these two historical phenomena—the widespread pre-meditated murder of infants by white mothers and the emotionally and psychosexually dysfunctional theories of white psychology—that are primarily responsible for

---

[39] *Ibid,* (See footnote 37)

delegitimizing co-sleeping as the healthy component of child rearing it has always been throughout the vast majority of the non-western world.[40]

Today western corporations have an added economic incentive to demonize co-sleeping as dangerous. This helps to ensure a ready market for the expanding array of infant accessories from cribs and mobiles, to surveillance cameras and electronic baby monitors. While this type of systematic neglect of infants has long been standard in european societies, for Black mothers and fathers to follow this approach to childrearing is tantamount to an act of cultural genocide. As Black fathers, we must understand that the Afrikan culture that normalized the practice of securely tying infants to the backs of their mothers so that they could be psychologically attuned to the rhythms of their mother's heartbeat (a practice that has demonstrable positive benefits in inducing calm, safe sleep) would never condone the idea that our babies should sleep in a separate room. In this regard co-sleeping should be looked at as not only a commitment to natural methods of childrearing but a divorce from a consumerist fueled model of dealing with newborns that places monetary profits above the health and sustenance of the family unit.[41]

We should cherish each moment we get to wake up next to our babies as inspiration for us to live more disciplined and ordered lives. With the corrosive influence of work schedules, media distractions,

---

[40] "Researchers observed that SIDs [sudden infant death syndrome] is lowest in cultures where co-sleeping is common."

[41] Anthropologist James McKenna cites, "living in a western post-industrial nation," as a risk factor in babies passing away from sudden infant death syndrome. (*Yearbook of Physical Anthropology*, 2007)

social discord, or the next viral epidemic competing for our time and energy, it's critical each day begins with an early reminder of what really matters. The quiet breathing, smiles, laughs, cries, or the silent, curious stare of my son is a regular reminder of what really matters each morning in my home. May we all experience the power of this bond in our journey as fathers, one which is available to us all through the practice of co-sleeping.

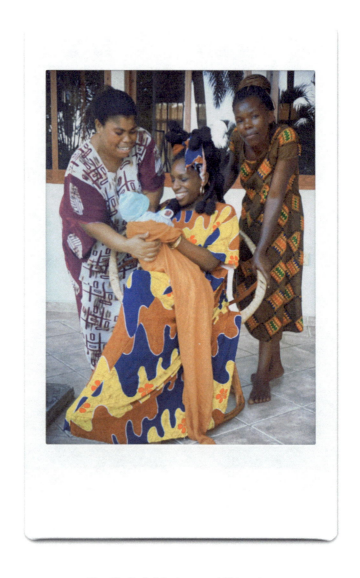

My wife, Dada Mwajuma, and Shingazi

Chapter 14

REDEFINING THE VILLAGE: INCORPORATING COMMUNITY RESOURCES

"Birth reflects the activities of God's work ... Birth is a central family episode that is met with a tremendous amount of joy and a sense of fulfillment because the expectation of a child is considered the highest gift from God. Thus, birth is a significantly revered experience for the entire community."
—Katherine Olukemi Bankole

Before our son was born my wife and I knew that the local Tanzanian community would be integral in our postpartum recovery. Attending the many challenges of cooking, nutrition, housework, and rearing our older son, all while getting enough time to rest was a formidable task, especially considering we were thousands of miles away from any blood relatives. Fortunately, informal, community approved institutions existed which could accommodate these needs. These caregiving institutions were customary, extremely affordable, and reflected the deep child-centeredness innate in all continental Afrikan societies. In fact, it is common for new mothers in Tanzania to spend 40 days on bedrest after birth to allow them adequate time to heal during the postpartum period. In our postpartum recovery two women (one an elder and one a couple of years older than us) provided around-the-clock care in cultivating an environment conducive to the holistic wellness of my wife and our infant son.

Mama Rose, affectionately known as Shingazi (Auntie), came to our home three times a week. During this time, she would cook breakfast for our family, clean our home, bathe our son and make trips to the market with our eldest son Mikey where she would purchase fruit, vegetables, spices, and other food items to prepare dinner. Mama Rose is fluent in Kiswahili which made her weekly visits an added benefit for our family, especially Mikey. Each day they would go to the market together Mama Rose would coach him on the appropriate Kiswahili phrases and responses to use in order to navigate their environment. This elder-child interchange is a signature feature of all Afrikan societies where the older generation is tasked with the responsibility of transmitting the greatness of their people to the youth. Acquainting children with their mother tongue is just one way this is accomplished.

Along with Mama Rose, Dada Mwajuma assisted us for two consecutive weeks (7-days a week). While with us Dada Mwajuma routinely bathed our son, prepared flavorful soups to aid in lactation, and was always available to watch and care for our son while my wife slept. Meanwhile, I contributed to this family and child-centered household dynamic by making myself available for diaper changes, store runs, preparing breakfast, and other baby caregiving duties. Collectively, we all organized ourselves in the service of the mother-child bond which is the basic social unit of all civilized cultures. But this can only be accomplished once we release ourselves from the social superstitions of our enemies and learn to embrace the sacred values of our people.

EXTENDED MOTHERHOOD: EVERY BABY BELONGS TO EVERY MOTHER

"It takes a village to raise a child." This is a proverb widely used by Black populations within the western world yet there is little serious analysis as to what it truly means and how it can be concretely applied to improve our living conditions. In order to arrive at a more functional understanding of this proverb it is first necessary to redefine what we mean by the term "village." A village is more than an abstract social unit. At its core a village implies a community of values. Sovereign villages are populated with men, women, children, and elders who share a common historical, linguistic, and psychological base. Upon this solid base, is constructed a cultural heritage which is then transmitted generationally to our children and grandchildren through community organizations.

By this definition "villages", as a social unit for Black people, are nonexistent within the western (american) context. The challenge then becomes how do we, as the descendants of Afrikan people, redefine village-hood in our lives so that we can utilize the community resources at our disposal for the edification of our children, families, and societies as a whole. A foundational concept that should occupy the center of our minds in this redefinition is the concept of extended motherhood or what Dr. Wade Nobles calls "multiple parentage." This concept of extended motherhood is integral in helping us as Black fathers to appreciate the role of community in facilitating motherhood and fatherhood in the postnatal period.

Under the institution of extended motherhood each child birthed into the community is recognized as the responsibility of every able-bodied, sane adult. Throughout history this has taken on various forms from wise elders (grandmothers and grandfathers) embracing their roles as teachers to the youth, aunts and uncles imparting life-skills to nieces and nephews, or non-blood kin generously dispensing with their time to add needed stability to our households. Whatever the source, communal relations have traditionally been held in high esteem within our societies. It is only with the violent encroachment of cultural aliens (whites, Asians, Arabs, etc.) that these natural modes of social organization have been phased out in favor of an individualistic concept where peers, or more disturbingly mass media entertainment, have displaced the community.

Ensuring that our babies are initiated into the communal model of childrearing as early as possible should be at the top of our agenda as Black fathers. This means reliance upon elders (blood related and non-blood kin) and qualified caregivers to help facilitate meeting the mother's needs. Examples of these needs include daily bathing of the baby, adequate supply of nutritional meals necessary to maintain milk production, treatment (hot baths and compress) to help accelerate physical recovery of mother in postpartum period, maintaining neat and orderly home, laundering of dirty clothes, and routine caregiving of infant to allow mother to get necessary resting time. When selecting individuals to serve as community resources it's imperative that we use our powers of discernment to filter out those who are fit to care for our babies and those who are not. Doing this will ensure a home environment whereby the physical and psychological needs of the mother and child are met without unduly sacrificing the cultural integrity of our people. Criteria for selecting community members to aid in the postnatal period should include:

-**High Priority on Elderhood:** If the woman assisting the mother and father in postnatal transition isn't a mother herself then the likelihood of a favorable experience is put in jeopardy. Elders are the repositories of skill and wisdom in our communities (Motherwit). Having them in our and our baby's presence will aid in the transmission of knowledge that otherwise would be lost.

-**Afrikan (Black) Caregivers Only:** UNDER NO CIRCUMSTANCES WHATSOEVER should non-Afrikan people (white, Asian, Arab, etc.) be entrusted with the responsibilities of nurturing Black mothers or their children. Since these people come from a culture alien to Black people they can only apply the beliefs and methods of childrearing which are native to their culture and destructive to ours.

-**Shared Moral Values**: The person selected to assist the mother and father must share the same moral values as the parents. This does not necessarily mean they must practice a certain religion or belong to a particular spiritual system. Rather it means they should be a person who evidences a child-centeredness in their everyday behavior. This includes gentleness, humility, ordered speech (no profanity), the ability to take initiative, and sensitivity to the needs of the mother and older siblings of the baby (if present).

-**Nutritional Literacy**: Assistant(s) to the mother should be well versed in what foods are needed to aid in milk production (lactation) of the mother and be available to shop for and prepare meals for the family. Remember these community resources are not only assets to the mother and child but, through consistent and intentional care, the community and is a contribution to the health of the overall dynamics of the Black (Afrikan) family unit.

-**Able to Assist with Yoni Steam**: Childbirth exerts tremendous strain on the female anatomy. Having access to herbal remedies to help in the healing of the body is crucial. Caregivers literate in this department are vital to physical recovery of the fourth trimester journey. In incorporating these community resources into our child rearing practice, it is vital to understand that biological bonds should never be used as an excuse to place our children in the hands of dysfunctional people. An unfortunate reality of life for Black people in captivity (the diaspora) is that many of our elders have learned to disown the timeless wisdom of our Afrikan ancestors. This has created a failure in transmission between the older generation and the present or, even worse, the transmission of the ideals of our enemies

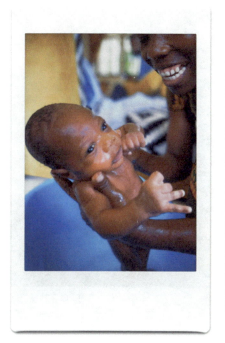

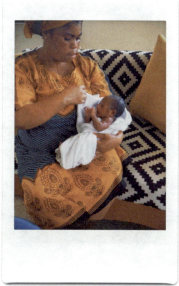

Mama Rose giving Jahi a bath.

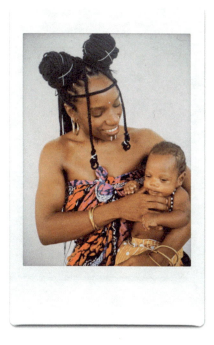

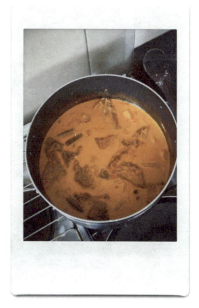

Traditional Swahili dish for lactating mothers

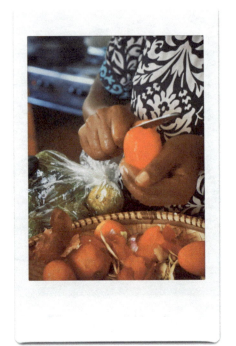

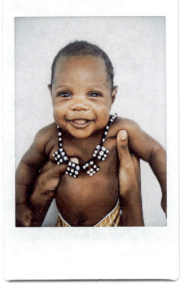

Jahi at 2 months

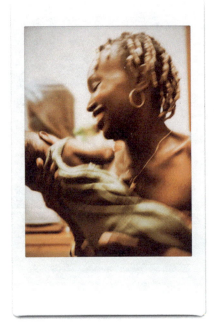

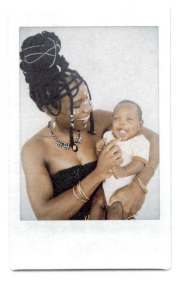

Jahi and Mama B

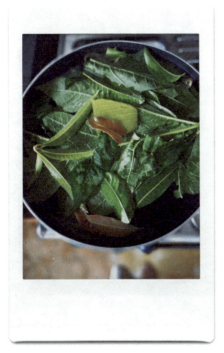

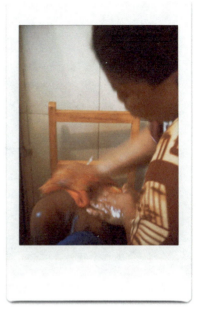

Dada Mwajuma bathing my wife
to help with healing after birth

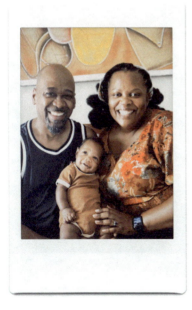

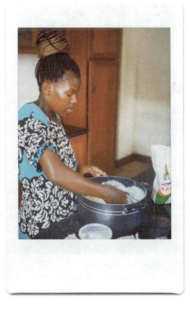

Jahi's & his Godparents

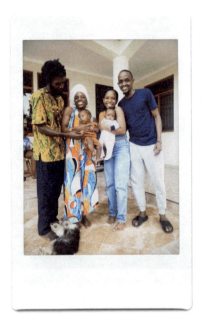

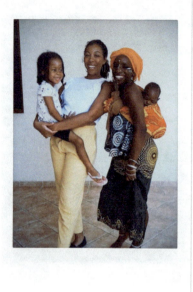

My wife and Mama P

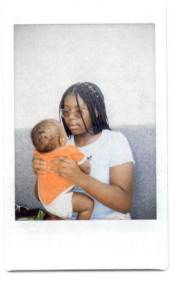

Our neighbor Mama Tyrin

albeit through the minds of our elders. Therefore, as Black fathers committed to affording our children the best possibilities that holistic, Afrikan living can offer we must develop the courage to have high standards of righteousness when it comes to the caregivers we entrust our babies with. In many scenarios, this will mean reliance on non-blood kin. Vigilance in this department will also ensure our children are provided with the proper foundation for the cultivation of intellect or as Mwalimu Baruti cites in his book *To Educate a People: Thoughts from the Center*, "The most important sources of the kinds of experience which form the infrastructure of intelligence are those which are the product of the social/educational interactions the child has with its caregivers and its psychosocial and physical environments."[42] It is the utmost responsibility of us, as Black fathers, to militantly protect and carve out paths for these caregiving resources to reach our families not only for the sake of our wives and children but for us as well. Bringing the community into our homes will make it so that we (fathers) are not stretched too thin and made to fulfill a range of caregiving responsibilities that can only be adequately provided by an energized and conscientious community. The presence of these elder women will also be a benefit for older siblings as their guidance will help them to expand upon their responsibilities as junior caregivers to their little brother or sister. Foremost, we are initiating our children into an Afrikan way of living that dismisses individualism as a western illusion when we welcome the community into our homes. We attain the highest height of

---

[42] Baruti, Mwalimu K. To Educate a People: Thoughts from the Center. Akoben House, 2019.

selfhood when we interpret it as inseparable from our peoplehood. Early prenatal care is no exception to this rule. Consequently, in our redefinition of "village" we arrive at a deeper insight: while it indeed does, "take a village to raise a child," by the same token it takes an empowered, spiritually-rooted brotherhood of Black fathers to protect a village. May we all become the empowered, protective fathers our villages need.

OXYTOCIN IN RELATION TO SISTERHOOD

As it relates to the variety of physiological changes that occur in the bodies of nursing mothers no chemical is more crucial to the formation of healthy emotional-psychological bonds than oxytocin. When this neurochemical is released from the brain of a lactating mother her aura radiates outward intersecting with the aura of her baby, the father, and those around them. In civilized cultures, such as those on the Afrikan continent, systems of social organization are developed to facilitate this transference of energy. From the Kindezi system of the Congo, to the practice of extended motherhood, and the general philosophy of child-centeredness Afrikan women have been the historical standard bearers when it comes to cultivating holistic, balanced, communal relationships. This relational maturity comes through powerfully in their institutions of sisterhood. When a mother is nourishing the biochemical bond with her child she is energetically speaking to the maternal identity of her peers. This unseen, hormonal connection is responsible for the high levels of cooperation, empathy, compassion, and trust that dominates between women in Afrikan social settings. That this bonding process is exclusive to Afrikan women can be partly explained by a recent study from the Proceedings of the National Academy of the Sciences which states that, "oxytocin's social bonding effects are targeted at whomever a person perceives as part of their in-group."[43]

This productive social dynamic is a far cry from the fragmented, individualistic relationships that prevail between women in the western world. In these corporate controlled cultures the birth of a child is maligned as an unwelcome intrusion which disturbs the selfish, recreational activities between adults. As parents rearing a child in Tanzania we have witnessed firsthand the socially bonding effects of oxytocin not only in the formation of parent-child bonds but also bonds between women. During an extended stay with us three months after the birth of our son a family friend reported experiencing strong sensations of closeness and affection with her 3 year old daughter. Despite not having breastfed her daughter since she was 10 months old she stated that the feeling was an unmistakable reminder of the "tingling feeling" she felt during the postpartum period. As she put it, the pleasurable feeling replicated the emotional rush felt seconds after milk is let-down. Here we had concrete proof of the revolutionary potential latent in all societies that elevate motherhood to a position of high status and esteem. When women are consciously aware of their potential to impart life to the children around them they almost instinctively link with other

---

[43] Pappas, Stephanie. Oxytocin: Facts about the 'Cuddle Hormone'. *LiveScience*, Purch, 27 Oct. 2021, https://www.livescience.com/42198-what-is-oxytocin.html.

women to accomplish this shared goal. This is the true contribution of Afrikan sisterhood to the process of nationbuilding and the scientific rationale behind the adage that, "a nation can rise no higher than its women."

Conversely, the systematic diminution of this "love hormone" in the industrialized west through the public discouragement of breastfeeding, the practice of traumatic birthing, and socialization into addictive behaviors of mass consumerism has led to a society overrun by crime and mental illness. Available data on the effects of oxytocin deficiency report, "Low oxytocin levels have been linked to autism and autistic spectrum disorders (e.g. Asperger syndrome)," with a primary signature of these illnesses being "poor social functioning."[44] So extreme is this culture of neglect that Black women in america statistically average lower levels of oxytocin in their bodies than white women. As Afrikan fathers, it is imperative that the environments that we protect are one's where sisterly dynamics between women are held in high regard. The first stage in ensuring this happens is encouraging natural home births, and exclusive breastfeeding by the mothers of our children and militantly resisting those social forces which either demonize or diminish the social benefits that arise from these practices. By following through on these responsibilities we will be doing our part to emotionally enrich the lives of our children, the mother's of our children, and the community mothers, biological and extended, who gather within the healing powers of her aura.

---

[44] *You and Your Hormones*, https://www.yourhormones.info/hormones/oxytocin

Chapter 15

DIETARY
RECOMMENDATIONS

From our earliest origins, holistic science has been the saving grace of Afrikan people confronted with the inevitable biological and spiritual challenges of the human experience. Whether we are speaking of the countless Oloogun of Yoruba civilizations or the elder mother herbalists of north america who worked to heal Afrikans torn from their native lands to endure slavery in the "New World", this deep understanding of the connections between the body and mind is essential to our collective survival. In the arena of perinatal health, the availability of highly nutritious whole foods during the postpartum period can be the distinguishing factor between a transition into motherhood burdened with health complications and one which adequately equips them to be the source of biological sustenance all mothers are meant to be.

For these reasons, it is of critical importance for us to cooperate with our wives to map out a health plan that will assist her in the physiological transformations associated with childbearing. Meals necessary for the promotion of lactation, healthy weight regulation, vitamin intake, and brain health should be developed and followed consistently in the interest of her and your newborn's long term health. Through this form of caregiving we are investing in the physical and mental wellbeing of our families while laying a foundation of wellness for our child independent of western medical "advice" or institutions. Some of the food items and herbs that are beneficial in the maintenance of the postpartum health of mothers include dates, okra, okra water, foods rich in Vitamin C and D, red raspberry leaf tea, sea moss, black cohosh, hot soups and wet foods. While some of the soups may include fish or chicken for plant-based mothers a vegetable only alternative is recommended.

OKRA AND OKRA WATER

Okra and okra water are vital to the prenatal and postpartum health of mothers. Prenatally the slime from the okra in water lubricates the interior of the uterus so that during labor the fetus exits the birth canal with greater ease. In the postpartum period the nutrient content of okra is also beneficial in lowering blood sugar, reducing the likelihood of heart disease, and alleviating inflammation associated with joint pain. In addition to being beneficial in water, okra is also an ideal ingredient to include in hot soups.

RED RASPBERRY LEAF TEA

Red raspberry leaf tea is a powerful herbal treatment to alleviate the intensity and pain of uterine contractions. The effects of red raspberry leaf include the strengthening of the pelvic muscles and walls of the uterus. Combined these effects make the labor process quicker. In the prenatal period, it is important red raspberry leaf tea NOT be consumed until later in the pregnancy (37 weeks or after). In the postpartum period this tea encourages fat metabolism, weight loss, and is an effective body detoxifier. Red raspberry leaf also has many beneficial antioxidant properties.

HOT SOUPS AND PORRIDGE (WET FOODS)

Hot soups and porridge are essential in maintaining proper levels of milk production in the postpartum period. Hot chicken or fish soup with carrots, potatoes, okra, onions, ginger, garlic, tomatoes and bell peppers is ideal to facilitate consistent lactation. Adding black pepper to these soups is also recommended to aid lactation. For breakfast, hot millet porridge is the perfect choice to promote healthy milk production. A minimum of two hot, wet meals a day is advisable to ensure necessary levels of milk production.

SEAMOSS

Sea Moss is justifiably considered a "superfood" due to its heavy mineral content and wide range of medicinal uses. Not only does sea moss promote immune health through its 92 minerals but it also improves metabolism, promotes digestion, heart health, and aids in lactation. Sea moss should be incorporated as a normal part of your daily holistic diet.

DATES

Dates are necessary to increase vitamin C and D intake, promote brain health, weight loss, and shortening of labor in the prenatal period.

All of the dietary recommendations outlined above should be adopted in a familial context, meaning it should not be the mother's sole responsibility to embrace a healthy, holistic diet. The complimentary dynamics that form the basis for all healthy family relations is equally as important when it comes to what we eat. Together, mothers and fathers must make a concerted effort to reform their diets to match these recommendations. In doing so the emotional and psychological connection between the parents will improve because Afrikan holistic science teaches us that the food that we consume not only affects the health of our bodies but also our minds.

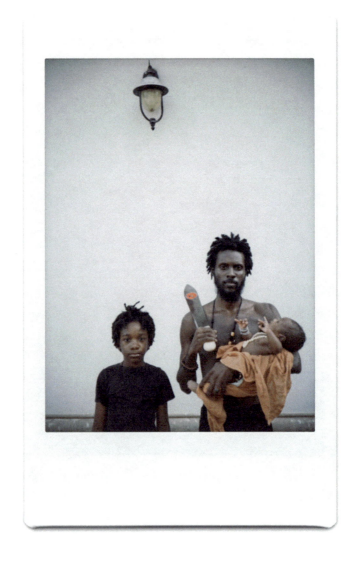

Me and my children, Mikey and Jahi.

Chapter 16

CONSCIOUSLY
PROTECTING THE
PERIMETER

Writing on the Fundamental Rights of African People historian and elder scholar Dr. Chancellor Williams observed that the Afrikan man or woman, "has the right to protect one's family and kinsmen, *even by violent means if such becomes necessary and justified.*" Under this constitution Afrikan men were also legally entitled, "to the protection of moral law in respect to wife and children—a right which not even a king can violate." Both of these fundamental rights allude to the protective nature of fatherhood within the Afrikan social-historical context and how failure to live up to this legal code endangers the physical and cultural survival of Black families. In no arena of life is this imperative to protect more urgent than in the domain of childbirth and childrearing. Allowing our enemies to oversee the birth of our children is tantamount to a zebra entrusting a pride of bloodthirsty lions to safely deliver its young into the world. Yet despite numerous reports of medical killings at the hands of white medical institutions, too many Black fathers have failed to properly heed Dr. William's words resulting in alarming rates of Black maternal and infant mortality without parallel in the so-called advanced industrial world.

Changing the status quo around Black childbirth will require that we begin to re-conceptualize the birth of our children as a matter of military significance. As with all nations of people, ensuring consistent population growth is essential to the social, economic, and cultural expansion of power. Therefore, we are acting against the most elementary requirements of group sovereignty when we passively sacrifice our wives and children to the trauma inducing-procedures of western hospitals. Dr. Mwalimu Baruti focuses keenly on this protective quality of Afrikan manhood in his book *Asafo: A Warrior's Guide to Manhood.* Derived from the Twi language of the Akan people of present day Ghana and Ivory Coast, an Asafo is the quintessential Afrikan warrior prepared to sacrifice life and limb in defense of his family. Traditionally, the defensive role of the Asafo would unfold within a larger social arrangement known as the, "concentric circle village model." Under this model, Black fathers (Asafo units) would maintain their posts guarding the perimeter of the village and providing moral and material support for family development in the interior. In this way, the father serves as the first line of military defense in repelling invaders. In the second layer of the concentric circle reside the mothers of the community. Administration of the culture, stewardship of the land, and the primary acculturation of the young would be performed at this level.

Finally, in the innermost circle dwells the elders and children. The elders would be tasked with transmitting the wisdom and language of the ancestors to the children and the children are responsible for the studied internalization of this wisdom for the purposes of future national development.

By abiding by these clearly defined, complimentary roles we would be equipping our communities to militantly respond to any threat, material or spiritual, foreign or domestic. Practical measures that must be adopted to protect the perimeter include:

-**Classify all information about your birth plan**: Military-mindedness is not just about securing the most advantageous position on the battlefield. It is also about operating in an environment of strict information security where the most vital details of our strategic aims are outside of the eyeshot and earshot of our enemies. When we assert the privacy of our birth plan we are insulating ourselves from nefarious agencies such as Child Protective Services or ill-intentioned individuals determined to deprive us of our natural right to deliver our children into the world. Attempts to accommodate these dangers by providing hospital staff with your birth plan is counterproductive as medical professionals abide by a cultural code above a legal code and laws are always drafted to satisfy the interests of the group that created them. Birth sovereignty is embodied in acts of militant resistance, not protest.

-**Withdraw from all social circles involving white people**: Transitioning into motherhood and fatherhood the holistic way is bound to generate opposition in those quarters of society committed to modern western medicine. Therefore, it is of supreme importance that we as Black fathers withdraw completely from any white social circles to ensure that the appropriate level of moral clarity and life-centeredness is present in our environment. White people are death-centered and they historically have viewed women and children as undesirable liabilities. Exposing yourself to their deranged culture severely risks disturbing the psychological balance the mothers of our children need (whether they know it or not) to birth our children into safe, spiritually balanced settings.

-**Cut off all dysfunctional family and friends**: Family and friends are earned titles in the Afrikan worldview. Prioritizing the growth and development of your family requires an ability to terminate stagnant relationships that operate on the energy of anxiety and fear. Tragically, we often find ourselves contending with biological kin in an effort to psychologically evolve ourselves. The permanent psychological damage that could be inflicted on our wives and children by complying with this pressure should motivate us to value our unique birth plan as a non-negotiable exercise of sovereignty. Trusting our own judgment and the judgment of the mothers of our children in the perinatal period is key in standing strong against this internal opposition. We must remember that family bonds can always be cultivated where biological connections are lacking through a shared spiritual commitment to our collective liberation. Lastly, this protective barrier must remain intact during the postpartum period as the delicate balance of forces within our homes that safely ushered our baby into the world will need to be maintained to make their first years on earth as emotionally and spiritually stable as possible.

-**Prepare an exit strategy from america**: While the aforementioned measures are highly effective in minimizing the external and internal threats posed by our enemies, no measure can

154

replace in effectiveness the solution of leaving the american landmass entirely. As a population that has been under siege in north america for over five centuries, it is a fundamental truth that every Black mother who gives birth within the geographic and legal jurisdiction of the United States is birthing behind enemy lines. This reality places us in an incredibly hazardous position that can only be remedied by a total separation from the nation that is responsible for our oppression. In this regard protecting the perimeter necessarily calls for a clarification of where the true geographic perimeter lay. For Black people in captivity that perimeter encircles the Afrikan continent where the first of our long lines of warriors emerged. Valid passports should be secured by everyone in the family prior to the birth of your child to help finalize this exit strategy.

Consciously protecting the perimeter should engage both your mental and physical awareness in order to resist any misinformation about allegedly "safe" hospital births. In this highly de-spiritualized culture we have become accustomed to narrowly focusing on physical health at the expense of holistic wellness which prioritizes the invisible, but equally important, psychological state of individuals. How our babies are delivered is just as critical as whether or not they had a healthy birth weight, were able to emit cries in a timely manner, were able to lift their head, or evidenced no visible bodily injuries. These cosmetic concerns overlook the violence of medical procedures which are designed to produce trauma. Therefore, when it comes to hospital births, "ten fingers and ten toes," is never enough.

Striking a harmonious relationship between the masculine and feminine in our homes means that we will have to reclaim our role as pillars of stability in times of intense adversity. In the words of our ancient Afrikan forebears, "a wife is like a flower and the husband is the fence that surrounds her." We will begin to actualize the immortal wisdom of this proverb in our lives when we, in defiance of western social taboo, stand firmly upon our fundamental Afrikan rights as the only legitimate legal code that can adequately safeguard our families and our shared vision for the future.

PROTECT YOUR CHILDREN

A defining feature in the overall stability of all Afrikan civilizations has been the high value placed on the protection of children. As the inheritors of the best of our culture children are charged with advancing the core interests of our societies and nations regardless of potential obstacles or personal costs. For this reason, both men and women should be equally committed to ensuring children grow in a nurturing and spiritually rich environment. The position of children in the innermost portion of the concentric circle model speaks not only to their significance to the community but a level of vulnerability meriting the most layers of protection. When it comes to shielding our children from external harm the most proximate layer of protection is that created by the village mothers.

Similar to the life-nourishing power of the amniotic sac that insulates the developing fetus from harm inside the mother's womb during pregnancy, it is the role of the mother to maintain the emotional and psychological equilibrium for their child to grow at a healthy rate. Meanwhile, the father represents that force needed to ensure the environment can be safely navigated without damaging this delicate sac. By asserting this role as the child's protector the mother is fulfilling her community responsibility and providing a powerful rationale for the fathers to militarize in their protection her. This mother-father relationship highlights a fundamental feature of all Afrikan societies, namely the degree of security that women are afforded is a byproduct of how seriously the adult population takes the protection of children because when the protection of children is valued so are our identities as mothers and fathers and it is our identities as mothers and fathers which equips us with the courage to protect our community against invasion by enemies.

This elementary truth eludes many Black families in the western world where the phrase "protect Black women," receives wide usage while deeper social dynamics that fail to shield Black children from the many predators in our midst are ignored. From firsthand experience on the Afrikan continent it is noteworthy how this phrase not only goes unused but for the vast majority of Afrikan people is unknown. It is the historically rooted culture of child-centeredness, skillfully preserved by the social norm of exclusive breastfeeding and extended motherhood, that makes these types of statements unnecessary. Afrikan fathers intuitively know the value of protecting Afrikan women not only for themselves but for their children and the community as a whole. When we as men and women begin to make a sincere effort to discipline ourselves to be mothers and fathers, regardless of if we have biological children, we are raising ourselves up to meet the needs of our children and our spouses simultaneously, laying the groundwork for truly sovereign communities.

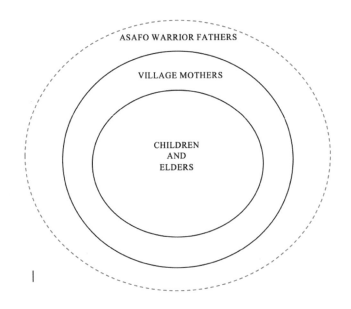

ASAFO WARRIOR FATHERS

VILLAGE MOTHERS

CHILDREN
AND
ELDERS

CONCENTRIC CIRCLE VILLAGE MODEL

Chapter 17

CHILDBIRTH AS AN AFRIKAN RITES OF PASSAGE

"Breastfeeding is the baby's holistic Rites of Passage into the physical independent world."
-Dr. Llaila O. Afrika

From a historical perspective, a key factor in the cultural integrity of Afrikan civilizations lay in their capacity to ritualize each stage of the psychosocial development of its members. These rituals, or rites of passage, serve the purpose of imposing balance and order (*Maat*) in environments that would otherwise be overrun by the forces of chaos (*isfet*). In this regard, perhaps the most glaring cultural defect of Black people born in the west is our completely dysfunctional psychosocial development, a genocidal process built upon an alienation from the most sacred ritual of all: childbirth. When european and Arab warlords invaded the Afrikan continent, kidnapped, and trafficked millions of us across the Atlantic and Indian Oceans to suffer the horrors of slavery the systematic destruction of the Afrikan family unit was essential. As Dr. Chancellor Williams notes, "the [Afrikan] family is recognized as the primary social, judicial, economic and political unity in the society." Central to the social unity of pre-colonial Afrikan peoples was the importance of ritual. Therefore, when our families were destroyed so too was our capacity to practice ritual. The Maafa of the transatlantic and trans-Saharan slave trade was most devastating not only due to the de-spiritualization of Black people that it set in motion but, more precisely, our de-ritualization.

Understanding that ritual is a natural, innate aspect of our cultural DNA (*asili*) as Afrikan people, our enemies worked tirelessly to obliterate from memory the highly elaborate and deeply symbolic rites that we practiced to replace them with rituals of their own. As a result, too many Black people today are ensnared in an alternate, european-managed system of rites where they have been trained to ritualize only that which contributes to their self-destruction. This alternate, european managed system of rites bleeds through in our ritualization of traumatic birth, child neglect, self-hatred, skin bleaching, european hair (weaves), abuse, indifference to death, the worship of white people, the hatred of Afrikan people, homosexuality, unhealthy eating habits, vulgar speech and thought, drug addiction, disrespect for elders, and consumerism.

At the root of all of these dysfunctions is a failure to seize ownership of birth rituals, the ritual that sets the stage for the rest. How could we not acknowledge the spiritual significance of childbirth or that our children were entities in the spiritual realm long before they emerged on this earthly plane clothed in flesh? Ghanaian scholar Anthony Ephirim-Donkor asserts this truth in his book *African Spirituality: On Becoming Ancestors*, adding that the spirit-self of a child is derived exclusively from the father, the mother being responsible for the blood. "It is the responsibility of the father to protect his offspring, because children without fathers, due to neglect or denial of the children by the fathers, render children spiritually and physically vulnerable ... Spiritual and physical bonding is necessary in order to bring about order and anchorage to children, and above all, connect children to the collective spiritual matrix." This notion of linking the child to the, "collective spiritual matrix," is a universal theme in all Afrikan-centered concepts of familyhood, a notion that we, as Black fathers, can benefit tremendously from if truly internalized. By adopting this perspective, we can begin to conceptualize fatherhood as extending beyond the important, but by no means singular, responsibility of providing for the material welfare of our children. At the height of our power we are the spiritual guardians of our children.

Our symbolic initiation into this spiritual guardianship role is completed through our psychological, emotional, and physical investment in child-birthing and perinatal process generally. When we are uncompromising about asserting our pivotal role in the birth and rearing of our children we are resurrecting an aspect of our spirit that our natural enemies erroneously believed to be dead but continues to breathe in our every move. Our power as Black fathers soars when we offer consistent, heartfelt encouragement to the mothers of our children that nothing can compete with the healing agency of her lactating breasts, supplying her with the psychological support she needs to stay the course. It soars higher when we diligently clean and massage the placenta, our baby's spirit "double", ensuring that all the nutrients needed to promote his or her growth are delivered before the detachment of the umbilical cord. We should cherish the biochemical bond reinforced through skin-to-skin contact and co-sleeping with our children, knowing that the blood that courses through their veins is of the same substance that circulates in the body their mother, forming a complementary pair with the *Sunsum* (spirit) that we have imparted. Our power expands even further when we look outwards beyond the confines of the family home, not in the direction of our enemies but to our Afrikan family in order to welcome a gentle, culturally functional form of caregiving that is the exclusive province of Afrikan elders. The constant supply of herbs, teas, soups, and whole foods help to round out the psychological comforts of our supportive presence with physical wellness, reflecting the importance of holistic health. Finally, our militant resistance to all white entities and social predators with intentions to destroy the peace and serenity we have cultivated within our family home distinguishes us as the first line of defense—Asafo warriors willing to sacrifice whatever necessary, including our lives, to protect our family.

Collectively, these guidelines (which were all discussed at length in the previous chapters) offer concrete ways in which we can *re*-ritualize childbirth and the postpartum period. If nothing else is absorbed from this book, this ritualization of the father's role is the core mission of what I call the Father Trimester. For far too long we have been deceived into thinking that divinity is a characteristic exclusive to invisible beings in the clouds, what the great warrior-teacher Dr. Khalid Abdul Muhammad called "spook-ism." But once we reclaim our sovereignty as Afrikan people, the first people to give birth, we will begin to understand that divinity inheres in those living organisms which are least removed from their primal source. It is my sincere prayer that the information contained in this book helps to illuminate for Black fathers the presence of this primal source and how our traumatic experience under the dominion of a savage race is but a violent interlude in a historical journey inexorably guiding us back toward our original state of power. In that moment, we will intuitively know that none of us were "born in sin," and all of us were born divine.

GIVING BIRTH IN AFRIKA: BREAKING "GENERATIONAL CURSES"

"No matter how others misconstrue it in an effort to make our Ancestors appear stagnant or backward, we are a future oriented people. Generally speaking, we abided by the Seven Generations Principle when it came to challenges which we had to rise above and had risen over in multiple lifetimes. The premise is that any and everything you do now should seriously be considered and framed within the context of its impact seven generations down the road."
    -Mwalimu Baruti

Among Black people living in the diaspora it has become a meme of sorts to champion the breaking of generational curses. Under this logic long-held dysfunctional family dynamics from abuse, neglect, drug addiction, or health crises of the body or mind are transcended in pursuit of more functional, balanced ways of living. Missing from this discourse is a thorough analysis of the social source of these multiple curses and how any refusal to address this source merely postpones rather than eliminates these harmful family dynamics. Etymologically, curse is derived from the Old English root *curs*, which denotes, "a prayer that evil or harm befall one; consignment of a person to an evil fate." A curse therefore can be better understood as a spiritual contagion borne from the minds of a malicious people. If we accept this the breaking of generational curses is incomplete without a corresponding break with the nation of people who first made this ill-fated prayer.

For my wife and I the gravest and most consequential curse that Black people face in the 21st century is the curse of our continued living in a nation (america) that has from its origin made our genocide their number one priority. Bearing this in mind we were convicted in our hearts that birthing our child far away from america in the land of our ancestors was not only desirable but a moral mandate. We meditated on the yearning of our millions of ancestors who were brutally trafficked across the oceans with unfulfilled dreams to return to the land that first nursed them and realized we had to honor their fight.

That I was able to deliver my son on the Afrikan continent gives me tremendous pause, primarily when visualizing what life will be like for his children and even his grandchildren. Afrikan centered scholar

Mwalimu Baruti expounds on the Seven Generation Principle in his book *To Educate a People,* describing it as an epigenetic process whereby each successive generation of children builds upon the contributions of their genetic predecessors with an eye toward total Afrikan sovereignty. As he succinctly put it, "What we know by fifty years of age, we should expect our students to know by fifteen years of age. Then, once they become fifty, they should be two or three times better at it, at understanding and practicing it, then we have ever been. The same should apply to the generation they produce and educate, and on and on, until full sovereignty is achieved." This multigenerational process of spiritual and intellectual refinement is deeply embedded in all Afrikan traditions which operate under an all-inclusive concept of family that links the ancestors, with the living, and the yet-to-be born. It is within this unbroken circle of Afrikan wisdom that all which is of great value to our people gestates and comes to life. From this circle, we also derive the essence of motherhood and fatherhood, which is to supply our children with the cultural resources to be the embodiment of our family mission and vision of what a human being should be.

That family mission should promote, at its core, the perpetuation of Afrikan living in all situations regardless of cost. Just as the Afrikan family is the most critical social unit in Afrikan civilizations, within the family the mother-child bond is most important. In fact, an effective litmus test to measure the level of mental and moral advancement in any world culture is to assess the nature of the relationship between the mothers and the children in that civilization as this will reveal its highest ideals of human behavior. For us as Afrikans the practice of breastfeeding is the biological and spiritual ritual that puts on display our commitment to progress in every arena of life. **We therefore should make it a priority of the highest order to have at least two successive generations of exclusively breastfed babies (for a period of one year or longer).** Following this simple directive will establish a firm grounding for a cultural continuity to take root and out of this newfound cultural identity will emerge the collective genius needed to guide us out of captivity and into liberation.

The outline of this grand vision faintly but powerfully comes into view when I ponder the fact that my son will never have to contend with the dehumanizing existence of being a minority in a white majority nation. As he grows older, when he leaves the house, his eyes will tell him that his people, and not theirs, is the global majority. The vision sharpens as we overhear his many caregivers speaking to him in an Afrikan tongue, structuring his thought patterns in such a way that his true Afrikan essence can be accessed without difficulty. Our son will understand that what he perceives, thinks, and feels cannot be discounted as marginal but must be respected as socially, culturally, and spiritually valid. Giving birth in Afrika has not only liberated our son, but our entire family, from the spiritual retardants that we all inevitably inhale under conditions of captivity. Growing up in Afrika he will look upon the abuse, neglect, and general disregard for life that characterizes the white west and see it as foreign. Just as my family, by the supreme grace of our Creator, were able to experience a divine freedom in abandoning the west that our ancestors could only imagine, we today should all be making the appropriate sacrifices to ensure that our children can say the same in remembrance of us. Abibifahodie to all the unborn Afrikan children who will build upon the work that we do today. We send our love across seven generations!

"If you really want to change the world, produce the children that will be that change."
— Bamidele

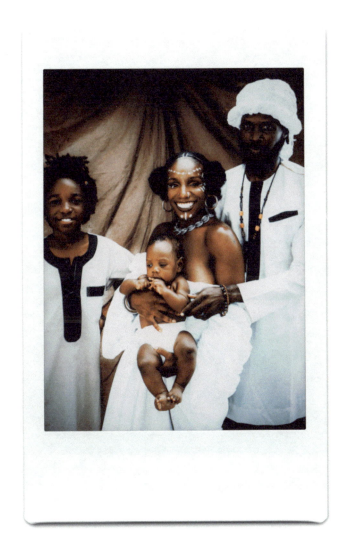

Made in United States
Cleveland, OH
28 May 2025

17307368R00094